THE ADVENTURER'S GUIDE

BY
MARTYN PENTECOST

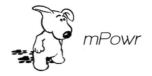

mPowr

This Edition ©2016 Martyn Pentecost
Original Edition ©2010 Martyn Pentecost

First Published in Great Britain 2010 by mPowr (Publishing) Limited
www.mpowrpublishing.com
www.celtic-reiki.com

A catalogue record for this book is available from the British Library
ISBN – 978-1-907282-38-6

Cover Design by Martyn Pentecost
mPowr Publishing 'Clumpy™' Logo by e-nimation.com
Clumpy™ and the Clumpy™ Logo are trademarks of mPowr Limited

MADE BY BOOK BROWNIES!

Books published by mPowr Publishing are made by Book Brownies. A Book Brownie is about so high, with little green boots, a potato-like face and big brown eyes. These helpful little creatures tenderly create every book with kindness, care and a little bit of magic! Before shipping, a Book Brownie will jump into the pages—usually at the most gripping chapter or a part that pays particular attention to food—and stay with that book, always. This means that every mPowr Publishing book comes with added enchantment (and occasional chocolate smudges!) so that you get a warm, fuzzy feeling of love with the turn of every page!

Join us on the
Celtic Reiki Mastery Adventure...

Free Mastery Training
with this book.*

www.celtic-reiki.com

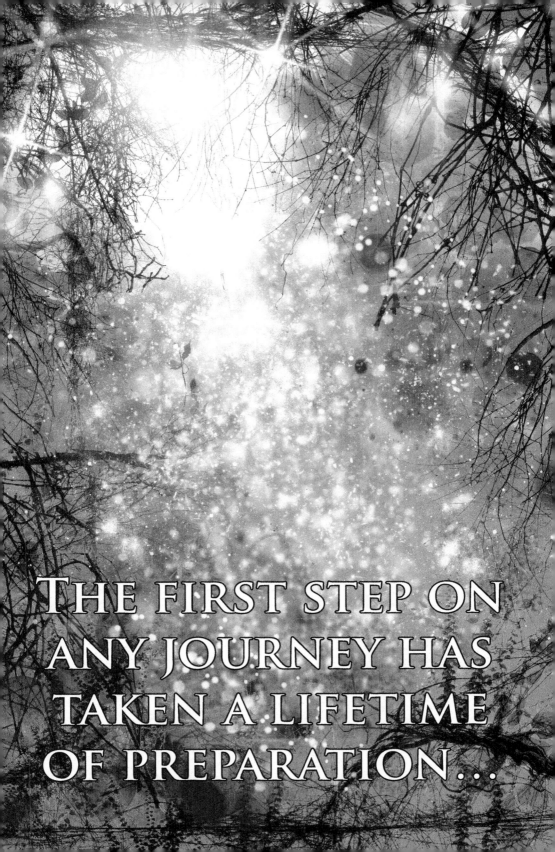

THE FIRST STEP ON ANY JOURNEY HAS TAKEN A LIFETIME OF PREPARATION…

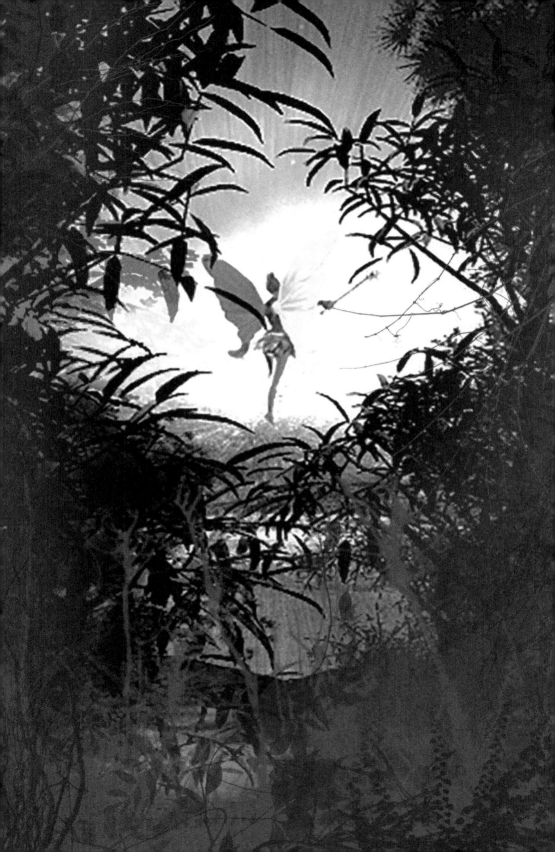

CONTENTS

Legal Notice

Across the globe, Celtic Reiki Mystic and Realm Masters are striving to benefit others through healing and personal development practices. They seek with benevolence and compassion to make a difference in their communities; to change the world and transform all they encounter.

In recent years their efforts have been undermined by a few, who damage the reputation of Celtic Reiki through carelessness, prejudice, or in some cases malicious action. This has led to the following restrictions to professional Celtic Reiki activites.

The practice and teaching of Celtic Reiki is restricted to accredited and currently qualified Mystic and Realm Masters. The certification of Celtic Reiki Master is based on a rolling professional development basis and must be updated every two years to remain valid and to reflect the current principles of our therapy.

Please be aware that when you seek out Celtic Reiki training, the only teachers/masters who are officially qualified to teach you are those with an **official Realm Master Qualification**. To check the validity of these, please ask any potential Realm Master to provide their qualification number and a copy of their valid training licence.

If a person offering Celtic Reiki training cannot provide these two pieces of authentication, they are not qualified to teach you.

Also remember that to practice professionally and teach, you must also be qualified. You can practice on friends and family, but any form of professional treatment must only occur after you have received your Mystic Master Certificate for practice, and your Realm Master Certificate for teaching.

These important regulations of Celtic Reiki practice have been put into place to maintain the integrity of our modality and the extraordinary dedication and hard work of our community. Every time a person teaches with lapsed qualification, or worse, no qualification, they damage the reputation of Celtic Reiki and fail to recognise those who have invested their time in learning the craft.

To ensure the highest standard of your training, if you have obtained this book from an online reseller, you will need to purchase the Celtic Reiki Book Bundles from The Official Celtic Reiki Website, or seek out an accredited Celtic Reiki Realm Master to train and qualify. For further information please visit **www.celtic-reiki.com**.

An Introduction to Celtic Reiki Mystic and Realm Mastery

Welcome to a magical journey... this first step is part of something extraordinary that will weave through your life and offer experiences that many will never know.

Celtic Reiki is a form of therapy that has grown and developed greatly over the decades. Like a tree, from seed to sapling, to mighty sentinel, Celtic Reiki was once a very basic tool that harnessed the innate forces of the Universe and presented them as the Earth.

Now Celtic Reiki has evolved into a deeply-acting healing modality that encompasses many tools and perspectives. It can be adapted and changed to the will of each Realm Master, and forms a multitude of treatments and techniques.

At its heart, however, Celtic Reiki is about defining the most profound aspects of life and sculpting Reiki treatments in ways that make an enormous impact. From physical, emotional, and psychological wellbeing, to spiritual growth, legacy and even business development, we can focus our Celtic Reiki perspective to form complex and ever-changing styles of treatment.

This life is fleeting; it is but a blink of an eye. Yet, within that minute fraction of time, we experience many moments. We strive for joy and happiness, we discover pain and trauma. We make magical memories and create problems that cause us to worry and fear.

These problems cannot be solved at the level we caused them, so we need to grow beyond our problems to solve them. Whether these be problems of dis-ease, financial lack, relationship issues, or family challenges, etc., we can only resolve each problem when we can view it from a greater level of knowing and wisdom.

Celtic Reiki treatment help us to expand our awareness to heal the challenges we face and develop new ways of living our lives with freedom and courage. As you learn how to conduct basic treatments you are laying the ground for unlimited potential in the future. You are learning how to transform the lives of others and yourself.

In this desperately short life, we seek for things greater than the spark we are—for the fire that we ignite. This spark is transient and insignificant; the fire is a beacon that can burn for millennia. By defining your life in deep and integral ways, by making a transformative impact in the lives of others, you are using the spark that you are to light the fire of your legacy.

This is not done with the wave of a hand... it is the investment of a lifetime. Something defined and redefined, adapted and honed into the artistry of life. As you focus on each and every area of your own life you will learn how to heal and help as the eternal Adventurer.

From childhood traumas, to the qualities that cause us to explode with passionate fervour, overcoming superstition and the mechanisms of authority control that bind us, to discovering the innate cycles, flows and secrets that power our Universe, you will learn many different ways of focusing the healing and strengthening power of Celtic Reiki.

You will explore our world and beyond; the moon and stars, the indigenous cultures and traditions of our world, and aspects of the Universe that many fail to know. And all this will take place in a very special learning, treatment, and teaching environment... The Realms.

This book and the others in this series form the foundations to a vast online environment—The Celtic Reiki Realm Mastery Home Experience. This labyrinthine resource will offer many hours of video training, audio experiences, sweeping soundscapes, visually stunning environments and further texts, which all weave together into the only accredited Celtic Reiki qualification available.

When you train and qualify as a Mystic Master, you will be able to conduct professional Celtic Reiki Consultations and Treatments. When you progress to the degree of Realm Master, you will be able to mentor and teach others, using the Home Experience resources.

These are more than just a website; the Realms act as anchors to a deeply personal and transformative journey; one that will release many mysteries and adventures. From Romanknowes to The Furthest Ocean and beyond, you'll be guided on a amazing voyage into your own psyche; discover your Core-Self—who you truly are and the the life you were born to live.

THE ADVENTURE BEGINS...

The Adventurer stood on the crest of a hill and surveyed the ancient forest that lay before him. The various hues of green extended towards the horizon, with the conscientiousness of a delicately sewn patchwork quilt. This place of tree and elf and the horned one was all at once exciting and frightening. For the forest was not of our world, and the way of things under its canopy seem strange and mysterious, yet oddly alluring to the intrepid heart.

He sat for a moment and relished the warmth of the sun on his face. Tilting his head he attempted to position his face so that it soaked up the greatest amount of warmth. He would miss the sun; its light and heat and life.

"Oh Grandmother Sun!" He whispered under his breath. "You are so beautiful and radiant, I wonder how I must seem to you? I imagine that I am small and insignificant under your mighty gaze."

A voice in his head replied, leaving the Adventurer all at once shocked, and amazed.

"My light takes all but eight minutes to travel across the dark vastness of space to reach your eyes. So when you look at me, you do not see me as I am, but how I was. No matter where you look, or listen, or touch, you are reaching out into the past to create a sense of how things were. As to what they are now; that is the realm of imagination and desire."

He sat, staring at the forest for the longest time and pondering the wisdom he had heard within himself. If this were true, how could he ever know the way things are now? Was he destined to live a life in the past, when he so desperately yearned for the experiences of the future? Was this forest old because of the age of time or merely the age of perception?

"How are you able to answer my questions?" He asked as he snapped back from his internal contemplations.

"My answers are in the light!" She replied.

He sat a moment more before asking, "If the answers are in the light and it takes eight minutes to get from you to me, how do you answer so quickly and how can you hear my words when I speak in but a whisper?"

"You asked how I view you. Well, our perspectives are very different." She continued, "You live in a world where light travels and flows from here to there from this moment to that moment. Yet, this is not my perception of the way of things."

There was a brief silence that caused him to look towards the sky, before the voice returned.

"The light that shines from me travels so fast that time itself, simply stops. Without time, there is no way of defining space, because this point here exists at the same moment as that point there. So, my surface and the surface of your face exist at the same point in time and space in the perspective of light; they are just different states of being"

He reflected on this for a while, until his thoughts were interrupted, once again, by the voice.

"If you perceive the world through your physical senses you will always be looking into what was, however, as soon as

EnergyLore

The faster an object travels the slower time becomes, according to Einstein's Theory of Relativity. When the speed of light is reached, time stops completely. Therefore, from the perspective of light (energy) there is no time and no means of recognising differences in spatial terms. To create measurement in energy, we define the 'state' of energy as being the parameter most suitable to encapsulate light from an Energy Lore perspective.

you shift your awareness to another state of perception, you know things as they are and can transcend time and space!"

The voice faded into silence, leaving the Adventurer to his questions.

As the Adventurer made his way down the hill, heading in the direction of the forest, he noticed how the sunlight was reflected from the leaves and trunks of each tree. A gentle, summer breeze caressed the branches, scattering light and creating dynamic, shifting patterns of green from lime to olive to emerald.

The Adventurer stopped and watched this kaleidoscope of shape and movement; patterns ever-flowing into one another, never still enough to discern an individual twig or leaf. In many ways these patterns mirrored the thoughts in his mind,

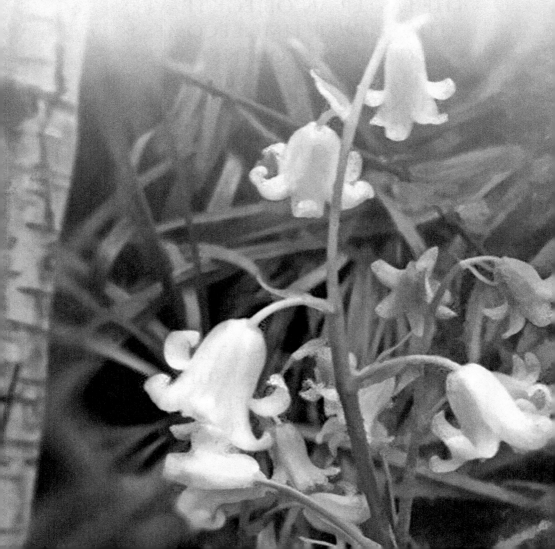

which remained just out of reach and never really coalesced into anything more than vague and distant concepts.

"If light is a series of different states of energy, sprawling out into infinity," he thought to himself, "then what makes one leaf different to another, apart from a difference in state?"
The gentle zephyr turned its attention from the trees to the approaching figure and skimmed past his face with curiosity and a somewhat playful intent. The Adventurer heard another voice, whispering to him in the breath of the wind.

"When you look at the leaves of a tree, you are witnessing a dance of light - a place where the physical world touches what lies beyond the physical world! Just as each tree reaches upwards to the source and the spirit of all things, you too have the ability to experience what exists beyond your awareness of the world."

The Adventurer was puzzled by this and quietly explained that he did not understand, so that only the wind might hear.

"There is energy that exists in many contrasting states and perspectives, and then there is the perception of energy. When energy folds itself into the illusion of separateness, it experiences the self as a spark of consciousness – you are that consciousness – the flicker of experience where the physical world of space and time witness the world beyond the world."

"But why?" He exclaimed for the world to hear.

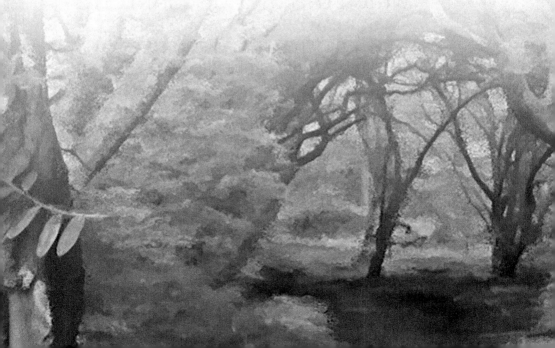

ENERGYLORE

Existing beyond time and space, defined only by 'state', energy exists without limitation or boundary, other than how we define it. Thus, energy is energy and there is no point at which energy is disconnected or removed from itself. So, shift into the awareness of 'energy in different states' and 'definitions of energy' as opposed to 'energies' or 'this energy and that energy'. This will help you remember that everything is energy and energy exists as a single interconnected force in many states.

"Because the Earth knows what it is to be an Oak tree, but he does not know what it is to be an acorn that awakes to the initial, fleeting moments of life; what it is to grow and break the surface of the soil with one's first leaf; he cannot understand the race upwards to the sun, or what it is to grow older each day, unless he forgets he is the Earth, that has known so many Oak trees, and becomes the individual Oak."

He approached the lines of trees that heralded the beginning of the forest, still confused and lost in thought. Upon noticing the protruding roots of an Ash tree, the Adventurer snapped back into conscious focus and looked at the trunk of the tree, which was so close that he could reach out and touch its trunk.

"Oh Wise Tree!" He said in the ancient Nuin language of the Ash tree. "Grandmother Sun told me that energy exists beyond space and time. That it exists in interconnected states of being. The wind speaks of 'folding' and energy experiencing itself from the illusion of separateness, even though it is one. Please help me understand, wise Nuin!"

The tree laughed, as is the way of the Nuin. "Little one, come sit on my roots and I will explain to you about the Earth and the sky and the magic that is in between!"

The Adventurer sat upon the roots of the tree, with his back resting against the strong, smooth trunk, and he listened as the Ash tree imparted wisdom that is older than any human or dryad.

"When you look out at the world, you see the Earth in all his magnificent mountain and undulating hill. You see marsh and sand and wide flatland. You gaze upon the tree and see an old wise thing that has lived for millions of years in kin and kind. You watch the ocean in mirrored calm and ferocious roar and gaze to the sky in vivid blue and velvet black with tinkle of star and fluff of cloud. You cast your senses into the world and you see separateness and isolation. You know here to there, and then to now, to then again."

The Adventurer closed his eyes and listened to the deep, resonant poetry of the tree, who spoke in half conversation, half song. The birds sung their cheery chorus and the Earth tracked across the Sun's gaze. The Ash tree continued...

"Yet the Earth is not separate from you, he is you; and you are him. When you look out into the world, you are seeing yourself through his eyes."

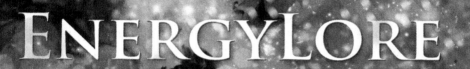

ENERGYLORE

If all energy is interconnected
and exists as a single 'entity',
every state of energy must
experience all other states from
its own unique perspective.
When we want to define energy
in one state as being different
to another, we habitually
separate energy into 'many' as
opposed to 'one' (that is 'red
light' and that is 'green'). To
define energy as a whole, yet
communicate the perspective of
a specific state, we use the term
'essence' – this encapsulates the
idea that the essence of Ailim,
for example, is the entire
Universe, perceived from the
perspective (state of energy)
of Ailim.

The Adventurer peered into the forest—it seemed peaceful and serene. Thin shafts of light streamed down through the canopy and twinkled on dust and pollen that glinted in the air. There was nothing to fear ahead—only wonder and the excitement of discovery. He lifted his leg and paused before taking a step… for he knew that with that step, he would be changed irrevocably…

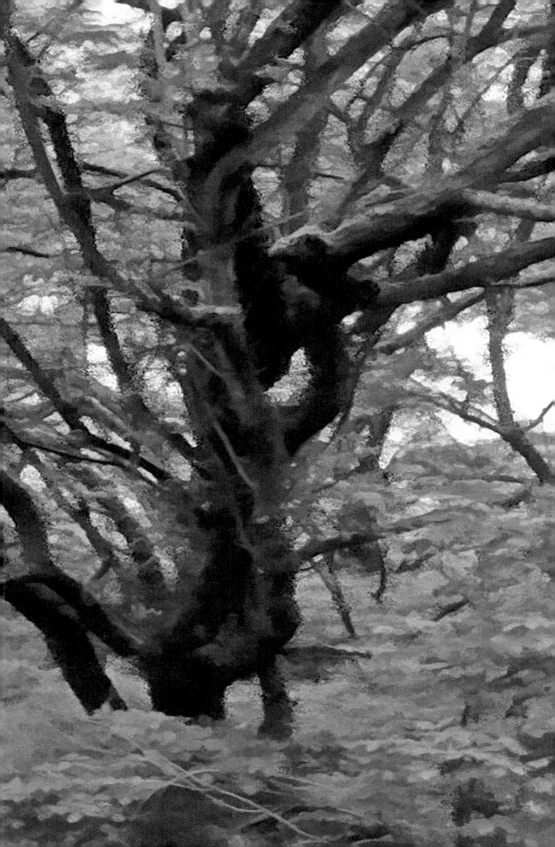

THE ROOTS OF CELTIC REIKI

Celtic Reiki is first and foremost a personal development method, by which, I mean it is a way of developing various aspects of your 'self'. This is an important foundation, because in actuality, Celtic Reiki is so vast in usage, methodology, and philosophy that it can become easy to lose sight of the main goal of the system.

I like to look at Celtic Reiki as a tree, with roots, a trunk, major branches, plus twigs and leaves. This analogy not only reminds me, at every moment, of why I am conducting a particular practice, it also helps to decipher how a particular tool, technique, or philosophy is situated in the big scheme of things.

As an Adventurer in the Celtic Reiki realms, this same analogy will guide you to find your own way of understand the huge array of contrasting, complementary and even conflicting areas of focus.

So at the very heart of Celtic Reiki—the trunk—we know that Celtic Reiki is a personal development practice. This means that everything we do has, at its core, the aim of developing you in some way. The roots are the history, philosophy, methodology and anything that is from the past; the physical ancestry or creation of Celtic Reiki. The main branches encompass the more general themes of practice, such as: healing (self-treatment and treatment of others), manifestation, communication, divination, meditation, higher-spiritual practices (such as astral travel, etc.), psychic skills and intuition, and so on. The twigs and leaves are the experiences we gain, the individual techniques, the moments and the actual acts of development.

Many people come to Celtic Reiki training, believing that it is a healing system, however, from the above metaphor, you can see that this is just one main branch of the personal development trunk. Many view Celtic Reiki as Celtic and Japanese in origin, yet these are just two, amongst various different roots. When all the roots feed into the core ethos of personal development and when every branch is grown from this same trunk, Celtic Reiki produces a very healthy spread of twig and leaf.

During your adventures in the Celtic Reiki realms, you will discover many different areas of practice, philosophy and aim; if you can maintain the tree metaphor in whatever you do, you will ensure deep roots that nourish you, a strong trunk that keeps you focused on the task at hand, and many powerful branches that can support a lifetime of experiences and joy.

Another aspect of Celtic Reiki practice you need to be aware of is one of historical context—let us call this the first 'root' that you will encounter on your journey! Celtic Reiki was initially formed by a single experience; a chance encounter between myself and the cloven Fir Tree.

You can hear about this event in the Stories from the Sacred Grove audio book. This was the seed from which Celtic Reiki grew and like any seed, it started its journey through life by sending one or two small roots into the ground to provide itself with life-giving nutrients. These initial roots were the concept of Reiki and a modern perspective of Celtic ideals, such as the Ogham, both of which we shall explore later.

With enough nutrients to grow, the seed pushed a single shoot upwards, toward the light. It was this shoot that would become the trunk, however at this early stage, the idea of personal development consisted only of healing and manifestation. Atop the single stem of this newly formed tree was a solitary leaf: eighteen *essences* or flavours of Celtic Reiki that could be used in treatment or for helping to manifest goals. It was this little sapling that was first introduced to the world and is still taught by many people across the globe.

The issue is that the sapling continued to grow into a mighty tree, with hundreds of deep roots and a massive canopy of experiential leaves. Very few know anything about the adult tree, only ever learning about the sapling, although every time a person takes the time and passion to find her and gaze upon her beauty, she grows even more and can support many more people.

So as you set out on your adventure into the Celtic

Reiki realms, you are looking to learn about the most wondrous, magical tree in the forest—and when you discover her from your own perspective, you will be able to bring your view of her to the world and show others where to look on their adventures into the Realm of Celtic Reiki Mastery...

EXERCISE ONE

To explore the history and foundation philosophies of Celtic Reiki, listen to the first extracts of *Stories from the Sacred Grove*, which are included in the *Celtic Reiki Home Experience*.

The specific style of personal development to which Celtic Reiki belongs, is collectively known as Energy Therapies, which basically denotes a therapy that uses energy to achieve results. The *energy* that is referred to is not like electricity, or light, or microwaves—it is much more subtle than any of these forms of energy. However, this 'subtle energy' does behave in the same way.

When we look back though history to ancient times and cultures, we see a contrasting range of beliefs that involve some form of Universal force or energy.

From Qi and Ki in the Eastern ideologies, to Prana in Southern Asia, Mana in Polynesia and Neart in the Celtic communities, this energetic force is often viewed not only as essential to life, but the very foundations that create life.

Even in more contemporary times, concepts such as Cosmic Force, Universal Energy, Organe, Source and God, are widely accepted words that describe an all-powerful, benevolent force that is responsible for all creation. Many people experience this force or energy in a very tangible sense, whilst others base their experience of it in faith and spiritual belief.

The greatest challenge for us is that this energy is so subtle that it does not register on most scientifically-accepted sensory equipment. In fact the closest we have come to scientifically measuring *subtle energy* (or Extremely Low Frequency energy) is through the work of Dr. John Zimmerman from the University of Colorado, who created the SQUID. This sensory device can detect vibrations of energy well below the usual limits, in vibratory ranges usually only felt by living creatures.

Most of the sensory data about Energy Therapies actually takes the form of qualitative information. This is descriptive feedback from treatments or observations from experiments, etc. The effects of energy therapies on plants, animals and humans is widely reported, yet this rich and diverse wealth of experience is not enough to shift the opinion of the scientific community in general.

Conversely, with such huge leaps of theory in the field of Quantum philosophy and other progressive sciences, it will not be long before a wider acceptance of 'subtle energy' and the methods that are built on it comes about.

In this guide, we shall touch upon many contrasting forms of Universal Force and explore with some detail two particular types of energy; Ki and Nearth. For whilst Ki forms a significant part of Celtic Reiki practice, it is increasingly important to contrast this Eastern philosophy with its Celtic equivalent.

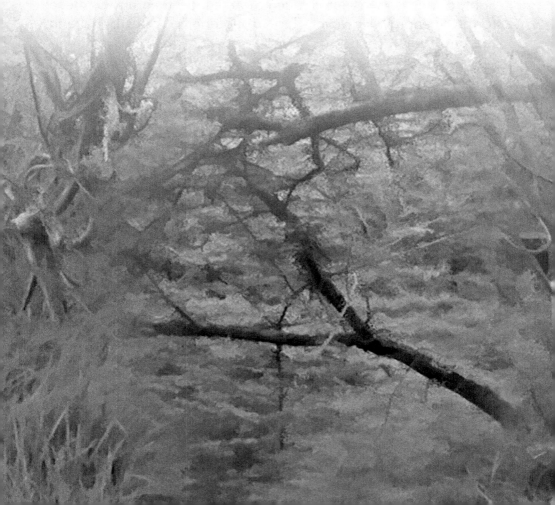

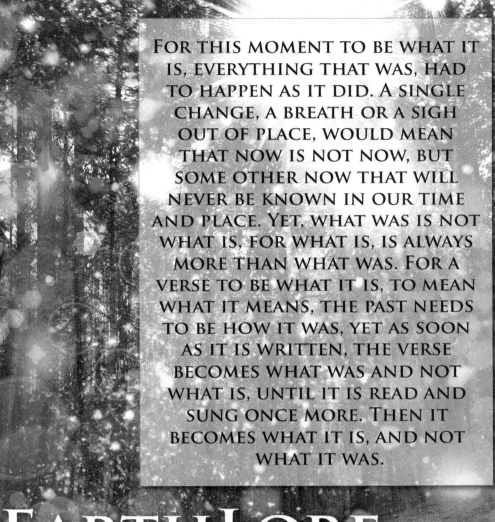

For this moment to be what it is, everything that was, had to happen as it did. A single change, a breath or a sigh out of place, would mean that now is not now, but some other now that will never be known in our time and place. Yet, what was is not what is, for what is, is always more than what was. For a verse to be what it is, to mean what it means, the past needs to be how it was, yet as soon as it is written, the verse becomes what was and not what is, until it is read and sung once more. Then it becomes what it is, and not what it was.

EarthLore

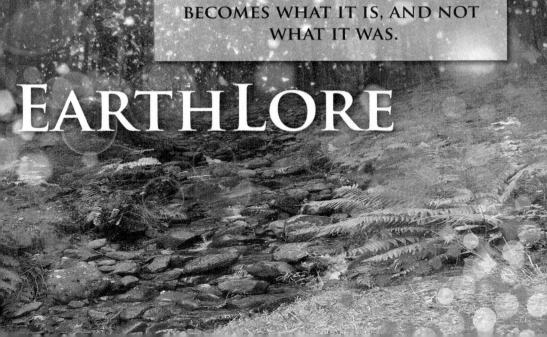

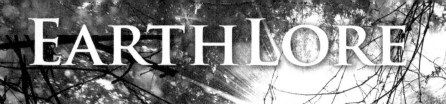

EARTHLORE

Everything we sense, by the time we have filtered, translated, recognised and understood it, is already gone. No sooner than we acknowledge it, it is no longer how it was. Therefore the present exists in some lost, unperceivable place that we cannot know by what we see, hear or touch. As time goes on, we learn to orientate ourselves to the past, turning away from the now and become buffeted by the future, by change and what is. Though, when we learn to experience our inner world of vibration and energy, we discover how to experience what is and what is yet to come...

THE SONG...

As the Adventurer moved through the woodland, the trees seemed to whisper in a strange and ancient tongue. These were not the spoken words of humankind, but unheard whispers that resonated with the very core of one's being. It were as if he could feel their sentiments as a vibration within him, a rhythm or melody that was not of sound, but of knowing.

This was the song of the trees; a lullaby, an anthem, a sonnet to the joy of life and wonder of experience that every tree seemed to revel in at every possible moment. As the Adventurer stepped over root and fern, there was all at once a familiarity, yet newness to this journey through the enchanted forest.

For the Adventurer knew that many had walked this path before and many would tread the same footsteps after, yet, upon looking down to the ground, the Adventurer noticed that the path ahead was not the well-worn track that one may have assumed was there. Instead, the path was untouched; as if this was the very first time it had been walked.

The trees serenaded of how every path that has been taken, by ancient stride and fresh, new intent, is untouched by all except the one who now walks the path. For every path is that of perspective and the unique viewpoint of the traveller— therefore, even the most travelled path is anew, with each and every footstep.

The ululation of trees seemed to soar from the low, resonant hum of the Oak and the Fir, to the high and heavenly melody of the Willow and Elder. It rose above the birdsong and the rustle of wind against leaf and took the Adventurer to an inner world; the place of memory and reminiscence...to a time that was...

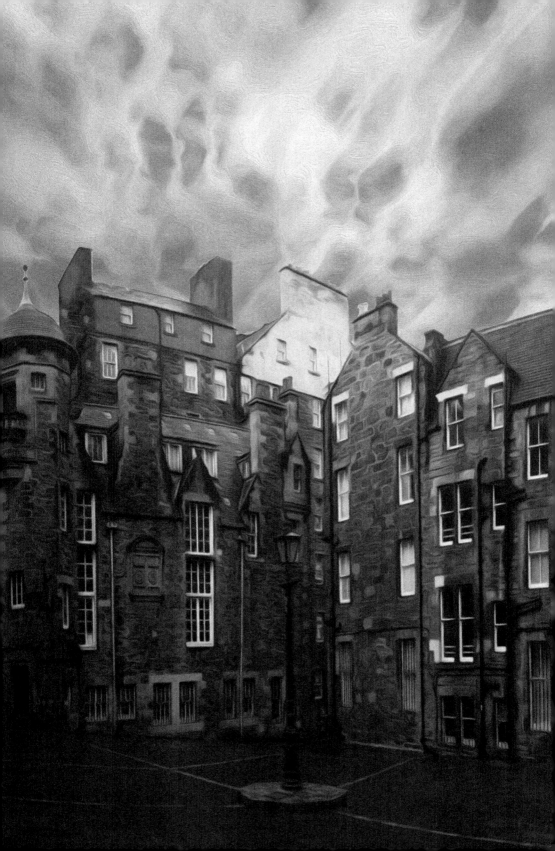

New Adventures in Ancient Lands

If you have studied any form of Reiki modality prior to Celtic Reiki, one of the first realisations you are likely to have is that the perspective here is very different to all other practices that use Reiki methodology. Rather a lot of outdated or obsolete philosophy has found its way into the ethos of Reiki, especially with the Usui Reiki Ryoho. Celtic Reiki readdresses this issue, to form a personal development style based on ancient wisdom, yet set very much in the modern world.

I am not sure if you have ever had the chance to read a Homeopathic Materia Medica in the original style, but if you have and you are anything like me, you would have spent half the time feeling nauseous and the other half, howling with laughter at descriptions of women who 'weep upon riding in a carriage'. Now, I am not sure if you know any women who weep upon riding in a carriage, but even if you do, I would guess that you can see how this description and others like it are hardly relevant for the contemporary world. There is a very fine balance between ancient wisdom that possesses a universal wisdom and ancient wisdom that remains ancient.

When I first studied Usui Reiki, I built my own perspective that was based upon the teachings of my Usui Reiki Masters. I had no reason to doubt the methodology, because this was how it had been done for decades. Yet, as time went on I noticed that much of the method and philosophy of Usui Reiki was just not relevant to the situations I was working with and, most of the time, actually detracted from treatments.

Over the years, I removed many traditional treatments and ideals from my own Mastery and eventually rewrote the

Reiki practice that I teach. I wanted the same for Celtic Reiki, which, at the time, was also based on the foundations of Usui Reiki. Even though the roots of Celtic Reiki extend back over thousands of years, I felt very strongly that our system would extract the most valuable wisdom from past traditions, yet be very powerful in a modern context.

This ethos can affect the style and ideology of a method in unusual ways that may take a little getting used to. However, if you understand why these changes are so necessary to our art, you will see the power that a change of perspective creates in the way we work with and perceive Reiki in our Celtic Reiki context.

If this is your first adventure in the Reiki world, then I welcome you and wish you many profound voyages ahead. Know that what I present to you is a heartfelt, much studied, body of work that contrasts with what is commonly believed, yet gives you a real advantage in the way you work with Reiki to offer proactive support and genuine value to your clients and students.

The most obvious areas where the Celtic Reiki Master's view differs from other modalities is in terminology and the concepts we use, internally, to perceive and define what we are doing at any given moment. For example, symbols are used in many Reiki practices to 'activate' a certain type of Reiki. Though, for me, this is rather like standing in a field, bathed in sunshine and saying, "I'm going to activate sunlight!"

The onus is not on Ki (of any form) to appear from nowhere – it is there at all times and in every place, woven into the very fabric of the Universe – the responsibility to act is with the Master or Practitioner. Therefore, symbols are used as a way of shifting conscious focus towards Reiki, as opposed to doing anything to Reiki itself.

When it comes to 'types' of Reiki, we use essences, which, as you will see later, rely on perspective, as opposed to being 'flavour-based'. Symbols do form a useful tool in Celtic Reiki, however, remember that they are a tool and have no power 'over' Reiki and their action is centred upon your contextual focus. In the time you spend exploring Celtic Reiki, you will hear a lot about perspective and shift your understanding to work with perspective-based philosophy. This very simple change of view by itself, will revolutionise your Mastery and heighten the success you achieve in your results.

To understand how Celtic Reiki differs from other forms of Reiki practice, let us explore the changes in ethos and look at some new branches of philosophy we can add to our Celtic Reiki Adventure...

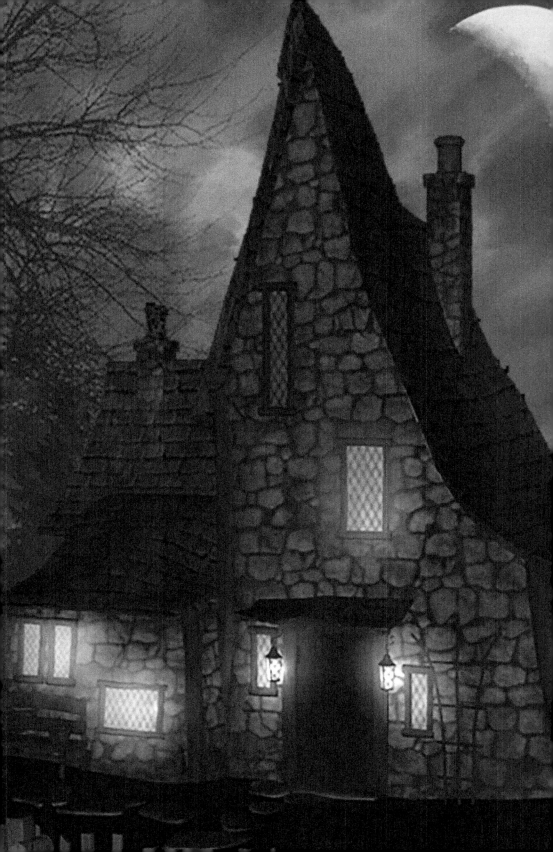

THE FOUNDATIONS OF REIKI

Historically, the nature of Reiki systems in a modern context, has revolved around the story of one man's voyage - whether this be Mikao Usui (the originator of Usui Reiki) and his satori on the sacred mountain, or my own experience with the lone tree - symbolism and ritual. As Celtic Reiki has evolved through time and the perspective of many, the need for tradition has become less important than the need for a valuable, practical system that achieves results in a contemporary world. In addition to this is the integration of this system into a much wider context. In the next section, you will see why this has come about.

This need has created a challenge in the teaching and practice of Celtic Reiki, because at the very core of our philosophy is the oral tradition of storytelling and ritual. This is one aspect that makes Celtic Reiki so popular around the world. The way this challenge has been met is with the oral tradition shifting to the way Celtic Reiki is presented through the Realm environments. Therefore, a system that is much greater in depth, historical foundations, breadth of knowledge and width of scope can exist, whilst retaining the simplicity of the Realm experiences.

Part of the process entails an almost complete break with tradition in view of the Usui facets of Celtic Reiki and a realignment of focus in the even older Shinto principles of Reiki. Here, Reiki is believed to be just one layer or perspective of Ki, which is much broader in scope than commonly believed. In this model of the Universe, Ki is a single, all-encompassing force that exists from different perspectives.

The initial philosophy of Ki is that it can be understood

from two distinct and autonomous viewpoints; that of the physical world and the non-physical intelligence. The non-physical perspective of Ki is known as Shinki or the Divine Ki. Shinki is the greatest wisdom that has ever been, or ever will be, for it knows all there is to know, except for one thing. The information that Shinki is created from can never be known, for as soon as you recognise or define a manageable 'chunk' of knowledge, it is of the physical world and therefore, not Shinki.

With all its wisdom and knowing, the one thing that the divine Ki does not know is so immeasurable in relation to Shinki's infinite wisdom, as to be all-encompassing and equally as infinite. This one thing contains all that exists in the physical world.

Shinki knows everything there is to know about kissing, except what it feels like to kiss the one you love for the very first time. Shinki knows everything about birdsong, but has never woken on a bright, new day to the sound of the lark. Shinki is the foremost expert on chocolate, but it cannot tell you about the taste and sensation when you place a piece in your mouth. Shinki knows everything, except what it is not to know – and it is this quest for understanding what it is to experience something without prior knowledge of it that creates life-purpose.

As soon as a life-purpose appears, it is known as Ishiki, the Ki of Consciousness. Ishiki is of Shinki, though paradoxically, it is also of the physical world. This is achieved by Shinki creating the illusion of separateness, through the 'forgetting' of what it is to be Shinki. As soon as this illusionary differentiation is made, Ishiki becomes self-aware in the physical world and sets about fulfilling the life-purpose from which it was created.

Ishiki is the most intelligent and wise 'entity' that exists in the physical world and it is also the most intangible. The elusive Ki of Consciousness is created from an illusion that flits in and out of space and time, like a butterfly. It is the energetic blueprint for everything that ever was, is, or will be in the future, from the perspective of every blade of grass, and star, and person. If there is the potential for something to exist in the physical world, its very core is Ishiki.

When Ishiki gazes out into the physical world, it perceives a huge mirror that reflects its own image. This image is made of many others forms of Ki, which are: Kekki (Blood), Mizuke (Salt), Shioke (Water), Kuki (Air), Denki (Thunder), Jiki

(Magnetism), and Tsuki (Moon). All these layers of Ki interact to create the physical world, according to the Ishiki 'blueprint', yet with such complexity and so many levels of illusion, wrapped up to create the concept of physicality, the reflection may form imbalances. It is the Ki of the Soul (Reiki) that acts as a bridge between the Ishiki blueprint of Shinki's life-purpose, and the different forms of physical Ki. Reiki harmonises and balances the world, creating a path upon which the solid world can filter back to Shinki and impart the knowledge it experienced along the way.

EXERCISE TWO

Listen to the first two tracks of Stories from the Sacred Grove, as found within the online Realms and make notes on the concept of Ki, Reiki and the other facets of Ki.

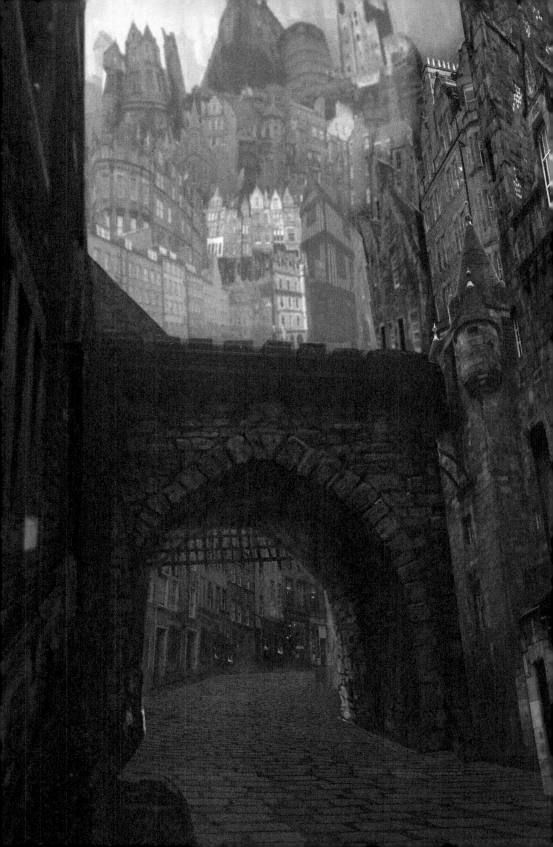

The Celtic Society

The Celts were widespread across much of Western Europe from around 12,000BC to 400AD. Formed of tribal communities, the Celtic title is one of language, rather than nation. From a Celtic Reiki perspective, this is intriguing, because modern Celtic Reiki is viewed as a lost language, not of the linguistic variety, but of vibrations. Of the once prevalent Celtic languages, only six still remain in the modern world (Scots and Irish Gaelic, Welsh, Cornish, Manx, and Breton).

The polytheism of the Celts (worship of several deities) is one of the aspects of Celtic society that, in our contemporary age, fascinates some and repulses others. This is most likely due to the monotheism of the modern world religions. In fact the Celtic culture was very different to our own and whilst it is often romanticised, it is purely through our own cultural evolution that we can look back with fondness at what was an often brutal, feudal era.

There is much speculation about the Celts, especially regarding their spiritual beliefs, because these were never written down. The Celtic tribes would pass down spiritual knowledge through the oral tradition, which kept it fluid and adaptable to the needs of each generation.

Much of the historical information comes from the Greek and Roman scholars who wrote down the observations of the Celtic people, and from the artefacts that are occasionally found at Celtic burial sites.

Many believe that women and men had greater equality and their spirituality certainly reflected this, through the role of the Goddess. There were certainly female warriors and women kings (as opposed to the queens of our modern age). Same-sex relationships were often preferred by the Celts, according to Aristotle, with relations between men and women reserved for procreation. There was a deep connection to the Earth and the natural world that was displayed through the sacred nature of lakes and woodlands (Groves).

There were also some rather unsavoury elements to Celtic society, with ritual human sacrifice and head-hunting playing a large part in cultural behaviour. Many of these Celtic Traditions had changed by the end of the Celtic era, with many converted to Christianity and thus most of their old ways (both attractive and unattractive to the modern perspective) became obsolete.

This evolution of society from the era of the Celtic tribes to the modern day is quite fascinating and one very important part of this process is incredibly valuable to our understanding of Celtic Reiki practice in the modern world. Many people do have a very positive view of the Celts and their ways; a deeper understanding of why this is can actually evolve your own perspective of Celtic Reiki and your Mastery of it.

Many modern philosophers believe that the gender roles in society and consequently, the way the hierarchy is structured, results from the specific values of a culture at any given time. It is thought that at times when a community is arable based, with the planting of food being the main source of sustenance for people, that women share an equal status with men in social and spiritual roles.

However, in societies where war or hunting are the priority, male roles are higher in status. Culturally, equal-status cultures are inner-focused, with importance placed on nurture and growth within, whereas in male-orientated cultures, the focus is outwards, upon expansion and growth beyond the community.

Personally, I prefer the perspective of social dynamics and evolution, which offers some rather interesting conclusions about the Celts and our modern view of them. For it is only through our evolution to such an expanded awareness that we can be so forgiving of the Celtic traditions; a less expanded perspective would indeed see them as barbaric and culturally unrefined.

Before we further explore the realms of social (or what I refer to as 'spherical') dynamics, let us examine what this process actually entails. The social dynamic is a parallel process, in which the individual and the community evolve in very similar ways. For instance, an individual and the community begin with a single person, fighting for survival in the world.

As babies, we are completely reliant on our care-providers for life and so, the only thing that is important to us at this age is to be fed, to sleep, and to survive (be protected, etc.). We have no care for others, the world, or anything that is not directly linked to our own existence.

Even our early learning is linked to our need to look after ourselves. The community also begins with the one – a person who is focused on their own survival in the world and will do anything to achieve that goal. This is known as the 'Instinctual Sphere'.

As we grow up, we become more aware of our family, classmates and friends—our social groups—and these people become important to us. We start considering their needs as well as our own and we feel love and care for those in our immediate social scenarios. Likewise, the survivors will come together to form small communities, realising that the many can cooperate and work better together.

These small communities tend to be very spiritual, polytheist, and focused on the good of the community as opposed to individual needs. Therefore, every individual in the group tends to care more about the 'tribe' or community than they do about themselves. This is the 'Tribal Sphere'.

This approach to life will often lead to the sacrifice of the self for the good of the whole. Consequently, this entails surrendering the needs of the individual and so often results in tribe members wanting to challenge the leader for dominion over the group. A strong leader will maintain equilibrium, whilst those who are challenged by stronger group members or rival leaders will often lose their power.

The transition from being a part of the group, to wanting to be leader over the group creates expansion into the Egocentric Sphere. Here the individual recognises their own individual worth over that of the group and this creates aggressive traits, power struggles and eventually war.

Throughout human history, the Egocentric value sphere

has instilled the attitude of 'me' against 'you' where 'me' is an individual, small group or community. This can also be equated to our adolescent years, as we develop a sense of individuality and personal identity. Many a parent with teenage sons or daughters will make connections between this sphere and the behaviour of their offspring!

The usual reaction to the anarchic wrangling between people and groups is to form authorities and governing bodies that create rules, regulations and laws. The idea of democracy is a concept born from the evolution into the next sphere of values, the 'Altruistic Sphere'.

The rejection of aggression guides us to form communities in the greater sense of the word, with the development of national boundaries and patriotism. The identity of the self envelops nationality and the ideology of culture is created.

We also see the emergence of organised religions, where people are asked to curb their aggressive egocentric natures through the promise of a better life or threat of some horrific outcome. Here guilt and fear are frequently used to gain control of people en-masse.

The result of this mindset is a rigidity of thinking—if you are the same as me, then all is well, but if you are not the same as me, I will ridicule you. This in turn creates dogma, prejudice and totalitarianism. This stage in social evolution is akin to early adulthood, the development of strong values and the beginning of moral fibre.

An individual may want to succeed, to be a valuable member of their community, to achieve in their career, family-life, or some other group/community.

When people experience guilt or fear, they learn to forgive themselves. This creates evolution into the next sphere where material gain is the main focal point of values.

The 'I want it now' attitude of self-gain at the cost of all else without care for others, is personified in the way memes are interpreted in the Material Sphere. Often the territory of business people, large corporations, etc., the attitude in this sphere is acquisition on material levels, even to the detriment of the care, health and well-being of other people.

People often become very materially focused in their late-twenties or early thirties. For some, this can last into their fifties or even for the rest of their lives! The need to own a home, create security for the future and provide for the family display the Material Sphere values in the individual person.

When a person decides to go with the flow and deviates from the significance of personal gain, they discover how to care for others, so finding compassion and thus often undergo a major change of some kind. This evolves them into the Sociocentric Sphere, where the care of others outweighs the needs of the self, therefore recreating the message of the Tribal Sphere, but (due to the Altruistic Sphere's influence) on a much larger scale.

The first people to expand socially into the Tribal Sphere in great numbers were those who lived in the sixties. The ideology of free love and Flower Power were the first inklings of the Sociocentric Sphere, even though initial sparks of these values can be observed in teachings of many spiritual leaders, such as Buddha, and in the formation of organisations that were established to care for people in a wider sense, such as the UK's National Health Service or PPACA (ObamaCare) in the US.

The sophistication of the Sociocentric Sphere ideals have developed significantly as we advanced through this social dynamic, thus, forming societies with ever-increasing complexity. The Sociocentric Sphere now encompasses many of the current philosophies in the *New Age* movement and, increasingly, within common culture.

The Sociocentric ideals are to ensure that everybody has a good life and that all are happy, along with the perceived role of custodian to the environment, all living things and the Earth. These values are often motivated by an underlying faith or trust in benevolent Universe/God/Source being.

Many people never reach this sphere on an individual level, although this is changing rapidly. Many people (especially women) tend to evolve into this perspective in their thirties or fifties – in fact it has been the speculation of many psychologists that if you do not evolve in your thirties, it is very unlikely that you will evolve into the sphere until your fifties!

The factor that creates expansion beyond the Sociocentric Sphere is the inability to control the betterment of our global community. When people continue to damage the environment and harm one another and there is a persistent lack of compassion, the Sociocentric values are replaced by the

Systemic attitude.

A person who actively works within layers of the Systemic Sphere will obtain, for the first time, the ability to actively work within the previous spheres, thus contracting as well as expanding. In the first six spheres of social dynamics, only expansion is possible, thus creating the illusion of a linear journey. The seventh sphere enables us to be aware of our contracted layers of perception and move between them depending on situation and circumstances.

The Systemic attitude involves complex concepts, the need to work towards personal gain and development, but with an innate care for others. The person who is consciously focused in this sphere will often have an issue with duty and will easily walk away from issues or challenges that prove to be too testing for the individual. Therefore the Systemic values tend towards lack of commitment and it is this need to discover devotion to projects and long-term goals that leads the Systemic into the Experiential Sphere.

This sphere also has the expansion/contraction ability, yet unlike the previous sphere, those operating consciously in this sphere will strive for unity and oneness. The overriding perspective of this social dynamic, is that all things are connected, with parts existing as facets of one complex overall system.

So whereas those working in the previous sphere will see themselves as individual parts of a system, this layer will focus on the system, as opposed to the parts.

The Experiential Sphere understands that the Earth is a biological system from which we are created and that we are bound to. As part of that system, the individual is also the whole. Thus, we perceive the beginning of the *many in one and one in many* attitude.

This creates the biggest challenge for the person working from this value set. The global attitude requires one who takes responsibility for all they perceive, because when you are not only one with all that exists, but the only influence over all that exists, the expectations you apply to yourself can be very challenging.

Being completely responsible for everything is the dynamic that enables people in the eighth sphere to become leaders, teachers, philosophers and guiding influences on other people. For the Experiential mindset views every person as part of the self and therefore strives towards healing the world, through self-healing.

When we look at the Celts through this philosophy, we see that the Celtic culture was based very much in the Tribal and Egocentric Spheres. In the earlier period of Celtic history, the tribes would have functioned much more in the community-based ethos of the Tribal dynamic. However, as time went on, the Egocentric mentality became widespread, with a brutally violent, feudal system developing and the increasing need for law and structure.

The last of the ancient Celts (those who converted to Christianity) would have evolved into the Altruistic Sphere and became part of a social dynamic that would last for well over a thousand years.

When we move to more modern times, we realise that most of the modern Celtic spirituality that has found a resurgence in popularity, is actually not based in the Tribal/Egocentric Sphere at all. It is actually a part of the Sociocentric Sphere, which is why it is such a positive and fond perspective of the Celtic traditions. The Sociocentric nature is to believe the best of others and focus on the happier, benevolent aspects of a situation or dynamic.

Indeed, Celtic Reiki was originated in the Sociocentric Sphere, based very much in a modern perspective of the ancient Celtic traditions and culture. Yet, over the past decade, the methodology and philosophy of Celtic Reiki has been adapted and evolved, though the Systemic Sphere and into the Experiential Sphere, where the ideals of interconnection and oneness form a practice that is based much more on modern principles than historical accuracy.

I personally feel this ideology holds the key to why Celtic Reiki has become so globally popular. As a Sociocentric Sphere therapy, Celtic Reiki captured the attention of people across the globe; however, with the evolution into the Experiential, there has been a sustained popularity when many other forms of Reiki practice and energy therapy have become remnants of the past.

The priority of expanding and adapting Celtic Reiki through the perspective of the individual Masters and my own need to evolve the practice have retained freshness, fluidity and relevance to an ever-changing society.

Of course, the importance of this debate is not purely of philosophical value, because the understanding of Celtic Reiki as an Experiential Sphere practice, presents an opportunity for each and every Master; by providing a goal and focus, with which to filter your intent.

Each Celtic Reiki Master's aim is to create interconnectivity, unity, and a 'sense of the Earth' in everything they do, keeping in mind at all times that they are part of the Earth and ensuring their practice reflects this.

To get a real sense of what this means, let us investigate how Celtic Reiki would be used by individuals and groups through the different social dynamics, as there would certainly be marked changes in the style, techniques, method, and ideals. These changes would not be from an intentional alteration of each element of Celtic Reiki, but an overall shift, created by the different focus and 'higher' goals of people (in general) working from the different social dynamics.

A group in a Tribal Sphere, such as the Celts themselves, would use Celtic Reiki for the good of the community or tribe, whereas, as they progressed into the Egocentric Sphere, the focus would change to, increasing an individual's chances of gaining power over the community.

A person or group in the Altruistic Sphere would use Celtic Reiki to serve some 'greater good', such as society or God. Those with a Material Sphere outlook would want to make money from Celtic Reiki Mastery and a Sociocentric Sphere perspective would see the individual or group wanting everybody to be made happy and gets lots of benefit from treatments, etc.

By the time we reach the Systemic Sphere, we see a radical shift in outlook, because not only are elements of all the other spheres present, but the Master or group will also turn their attention inwards, to focus on the practice itself. Here Celtic Reiki becomes much more defined as a living entity. She becomes a complex, living system that is not only about 'how many essences and attunements' she has, but how she can attain an internal 'beauty' and balance of complexity, efficiency, and power, that offers real benefits to everybody.

The Celtic Reiki that is viewed by the (rare, but becoming more prevalent) Experiential Sphere group or Master integrates into a single entity, where Master/group/Celtic Reiki/Earth are all one. It is a practice of definition only, where everything is a dynamic, bioenergetic, living system or sentience, that strives to understand itself through the methodology and individuals he encompasses.

This mind-blowing concept is rather complex, but the basic gist is that the Celtic Reiki Master who works from the Experiential Sphere, will view herself as a part of a larger entity – for example: the Earth - working through her and Celtic Reiki to heal himself and expand in awareness, etc. or the Universe, defining itself as Celtic Reiki and perceiving self-mastery through the sensory experiences of the Master.

The Realm was built from an even greater expansion of perception, so there is plenty of room for Celtic Reiki to expand into new spheres of social dynamic, however, with so few people currently working from the Experiential view, this is something to look forward to.

Before we move on, there are some additional points to remember when working with the social dynamic model. The most important of these, is that a person can work from different spheres when carrying out different activities. So, they may view their work from a Material Sphere, home life from a Tribal Sphere and spirituality from an Altruistic Sphere.

When they function from a specific sphere they will view the other spheres from that position only, thus cannot be in two spheres at the same time (unless it is the Systemic or Experiential Spheres).

People cannot perceive the sphere above until they experience it for themselves. So when a person or group in the dynamic of the Sociocentric Sphere comes into contact with a person who is using the Systemic Sphere perspective, they will see a Material perspective – usually somebody who is out to make money, without regard for others.

Alternate spheres have an affinity with each other through focus, though this is not always harmonious! A spiritually-focused example could be, a Christian (Altruistic) may view group a with New Age principles (Sociocentric) as a Pagan organisation (Tribal). And it is not only other spheres that do this—I have met many of a Sociocentric Sphere perspective that believe themselves to be of the Tribal Sphere. Here we also notice the tendency for a more expanded dynamic to frown upon the 'alternate sphere', below. Hence, those of Systemic perception may look down upon Material Sphere groups, etc.

To complete this discussion and as a means of summary, there is one final aspect that is rather intriguing. This is what happens when you apply the social dynamics philosophy to a person who is working through their Celtic Reiki Mastery.

Here we see the initial reasons for a person to work with Celtic Reiki are for self-treatment (Instinctual), though soon they realise the benefits for their family and friends (Tribal). As they treat others with success, the Master may develop a sense of power of possessing some special gift (Egocentric), and this is so open to abuse that they need to lay down laws of practice or abide by rules (Altruistic).

Eventually they realise that they can make some money from teaching Celtic Reiki (Material), but more than that, they can help many people across the world at the same time (Sociocentric).

When a Master reaches the Systemic Sphere, they view Celtic Reiki as a system that requires complexity to truly help the diverse cultural, social, and individual needs of the people they treat. This diversity needs to encompass, not only an historical context (vast ages of wisdom), but methodology (lots of different, adaptable tools), and philosophy (embracing psychology, theology, physiology, sociology, and so on). Thus, a complex and diverse system is born that is far removed from the simple structure of previous iterations.

Finally, the Experiential Sphere perspective is achieved by the Master and they look upon Celtic Reiki as the Earth, learning, evolving, self-realising, through the human experience of Celtic Reiki. The separation between themselves, other people, trees, all living things and the Earth become virtually unnoticeable and the Master's role takes on a whole new meaning.

THE EARTH AND THE STARS

Our Universe is a multifaceted and complex entity in nature and action that is so infinitely vast that we can never know all there is to know. The mysteries of this incomprehensible expanse are woven through the very fabric of life; glimpsed in the fleeting moments of our lives through the glimmer of the tiniest gesture or the most profound miracle. In many ways Celtic Reiki is about acknowledging and recognising these precious fragments of clarity, as it is about the definitions and ideals we place upon it.

The core philosophy of the Universe that is often ignored or overlooked is that it is constantly expanding into the unknown. This infinite entity consists of everything that ever was or will be and yet, it is constantly growing at every point. What is it moving into? What exists beyond the Universe? Well, the paradoxical answer to this is that there is nothing beyond the Universe, because as soon as you define what the Universe is expanding into, that thing becomes part of the Universe and is no longer 'outside' of it!

Therefore the important concept for our focus here is not what exists outside, but the process of internal expansion. This expansion occurs at every point of the Universe and thus, is occurring at every point of your being; physically, cerebrally, spiritually. You spend a lifetime expanding beyond what you were before to the extent that, at any given moment, you are more than everything you have ever been at every other moment.

Change and adaptation is a challenge for many people, because with change comes a reassessment of everything we have grown comfortable with and an invitation to be uncomfortable for a while. Just as our eyes become accustomed to the light, we are cast into darkness and need to find our way all over again. This manifests in many ways for us. Some people choose to stick to their current ways, no matter what, and often stay where they are until dis-ease and trauma wrack their very being.

Some adapt slowly and in the form of a jerky dynamic that creates rapid change and then long periods of stagnation. A number of people deceive themselves into believing that they are changing and adapting, when they are actually creating more of the same, or expanding only in one direction. A few simply surrender and release their connection to life, either physically, emotionally, or mentally.

In the context of Reiki therapies, I have witnessed these habitual responses to expansion, time and time again. From the Masters who create adaptation by simply collecting symbols or focusing on more attunements, to those who actively attempt to stop change by dogmatically clinging to traditional methods, in some cases without ever giving adequate focus to alternatives.

Energy, force, Reiki, Nearth, consciousness, thought, being, even the solid Universe, is always more, consistently changing and growing. If you are not mirroring this process, then you are enveloping yourself into what was and not what is.

When you gaze into the night sky, every star you gaze upon is not only further away from you than ever before, it is also further away from every other star and more expanded within itself.

Some of those stars are no longer there in actual space; the light they emitted millions of years ago has taken such an age to arrive here in terms of physical, sensory perception, that you are actually seeing ghostly images of some ancient time that no longer exists.

Apply this same ethos to energy arts and we see that without the frequent challenge of 'actual' evolution (as opposed to simple addition) we can end up working with memories, echoes, and the afterimage left in our eyes when the light has long since disappeared.

Indeed, the Viridian philosophies that I personally work with suggest that Reiki, as we know it, no longer exists within our current time, but it is the memory of it that we work with in treatment and technique. It was this realisation that led me on my own personal journey to revolutionise Celtic Reiki and what

I call vReiki.

The legacy I leave every Master with, is that of expanding their own practice with the same level of adaptation and change as is necessary to remain 'in potential' in the Universe. And by this, I mean that if your therapy only exists in what you knew last month, last week, yesterday or this morning, then it no longer has the potential to achieve everything you require of it in this moment and this moment and this…

The analogy that the stars provide us with is so profound in many ways, for when we understand that a star has a physical reality and a physical illusion, we realise so many parallels with our Earthly existence.

For here on Earth, how much is real and how much is illusion? Is the ground beneath your feet what is, or what was once was? Are you only the physical body and the thoughts it creates, in which case, when did you stop being that apple or piece of chocolate and start being the physical body? Are you a solid receptacle for a spirit or soul? Are you energy interacting as the physical world? When you look in the mirror, does the reflection show you who you are, who you were, or is it an illusion of light?

From my earliest memories I can remember being defined by others. A good proportion of these definitions were about my physical body, be it 'too fat', 'too thin', 'too tall', 'feet too big'. There were also 'behavioural' definitions which were sometimes in the moment: 'you are talented' or 'you're a fat fool'. And on other occasions, they were out of the moment: 'you have always let me down' or 'you will never succeed'.

The fact is that I believed these definitions to be true for such a long time, until I realised that these were not definitions of me, but actually the perceptions of others. The physical definitions are relative and the behavioural definitions said more about the other people than they did about me. Yet, even this was only another layer of truth, because all these things are actually thoughts that are encoded as memories – they are light from stars that may not even exist and may have never existed in the lifetime of this body.

So, am I the reflection in the mirror? Am I the thoughts that consciously define me as the source of that reflection? Could I be the light that bounces from physical body to polished glass? Am I words on a page, or thoughts in your own mind?

If I look into a mirror and believe myself to be 'too fat', am I defining myself how I am, how I was, or am I the definition of a dietician in 1982? Have I stored those parameters up for many years, simply to repeat them now, or has that definition just taken a while to get here?

For me the truth is far more profound than any of these questions can offer in solution. For in recent years I realise that from moment to moment I am not the Earth, gazing at the spectral and ghostly memories of stars – I am the starlight, experiencing this moment through the consciousness of Earth.

Several years ago, when I began to develop facial wrinkles, like most people, I really disliked the 'signs of aging'. I soon realised that this was a definition created by others to create a reaction.

What I was actually experiencing was the natural life cycle of a human body. I was one of the privileged few to actually see, touch and feel one of the most precious gifts we can ever know. Life. Not conception, or birth, or beginning, but life, in a beautiful, complex dance of wisdom and experience. I was getting the opportunity to witness every smile this body has ever smiled, every tear of sorrow and joy, every mischievous raise of an eyebrow and every wide-eyed gaze of wonder.

It was at this moment that I knew I was not this body, but the something other than this body; an incomprehensible, indefinable, benevolent force that was peering into the physical world and moving beyond the limitations and trivialities of society to experience the wonder of a body.

A body, doing what bodies do, so that I could be there to notice. You see, this body smiled all those smiles, shed all those tears, and mischievously raised eyebrows in all directions, not for some random and coincidental collection of transitory reasons, but so that I could look through those eyes to know what it was to be so blessed and privileged in that moment.

When you truly grasp this concept you realise that you have a choice… Are you a Celtic Reiki Master who looks back to the past and harks for a simpler time when all was good with the world? Are you a Celtic Reiki Master that uses ancient philosophy in a modern perspective to create something new? Or are you ancient wisdom, as a thought, a spark, presented with the chance to experience a moment of wondrous potential through a physical body and the conscious awareness it offers?

For we all have the choice to view ourselves as the Earth and being of the Earth, or of being starlight, born of a long forgotten sun that may no longer exist, but given the chance to be experienced through the eyes of another who chances a look in our direction.

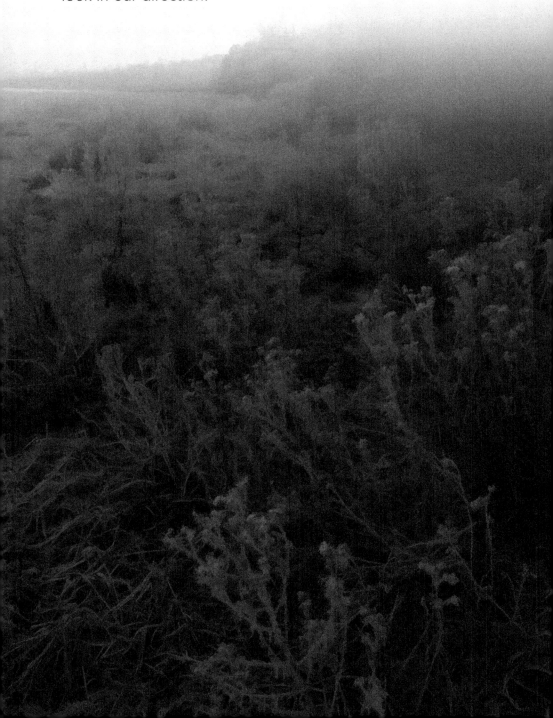

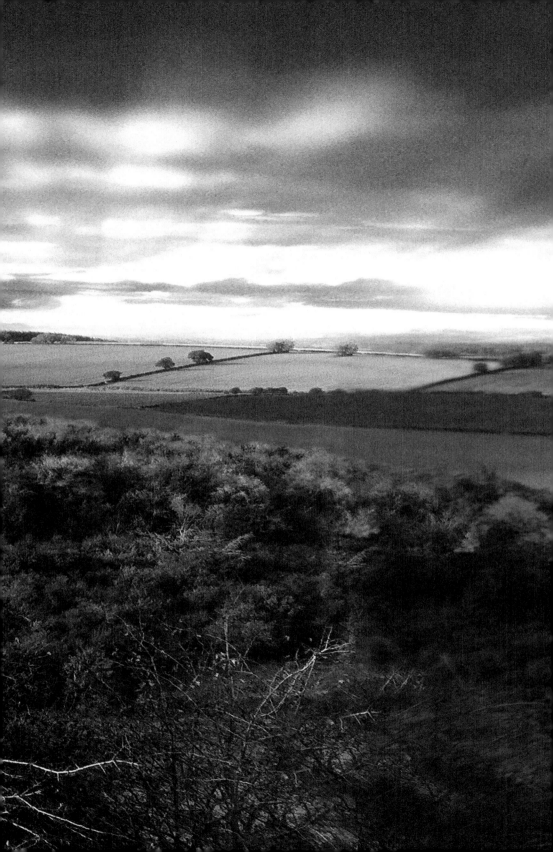

Nearth: A Celtic Reimagining

Almost every civilisation that has a close connection to the natural world realises one innate spark of wisdom: being healthy and happy is the natural state of living. Dis-ease, sadness, pain, lack, and so on all come about when we are misaligned with the Earth and the natural forces of the Universe.

Our ancestors were certainly much more in tune with the Earth and natural unity of all things. Just as birds navigate using magnetic fields and animals when a thunderstorm approaches, our ancestors could navigate the oceans by studying the patterns of waves and divine for underground water sources, using their intuition only. Even in our contemporary world there are stories of aboriginal Australians who can disguise themselves as trees, or Native American Shamans who can 'cloudburst'.

It is very likely that the Celts lived their lives through a deep connection to the Earth. Their alignment with the cycles and rhythms of their surrounding ecosystem was essential, not only to farming, foraging and hunting, but also when travelling or finding a base for their communities, etc.

To a great extent, we have lost this connection and spend much of our time convincing ourselves that the world is there to serve our own needs. We live and work in glass and concrete, with jobs that are often there for their own sake. Ask most city dwellers where the nearest fresh water could be located and they would be unable to tell you, even though water is an essential need.

As humankind evolved to adapt our environments to our needs, we left behind many of the hardships and challenges that the Celts and other indigenous cultures faced. However, we also lost many of the inherent gifts that naturally enhance our lives through the health and happiness they provide. It is one of these gifts that we are rediscovering through means such as the Reiki therapies and other energy arts. For as we reconnect to our ability to sense subtle vibrations of energy, we rediscover the connections that our ancestors had.

Over the years, many Masters have explained to me that their perspective of Celtic Reiki is what they can best describe as Nearth (or Neart); the life-force, believed to be a connective thread through the Celtic traditions.

Some Masters believe Celtic Reiki to be a rediscovery of Nearth—a Reiki of the Celts, whilst others believe it is a contemporary equivalent—the modern version of a Universal energy or life-force. Personally, I believe that each Master needs to find their own answers regarding the question of whether Celtic Reiki is an ancient Japanese force, redefined in a Celtic perspective, the reconnection to a Celtic life-force, or a new form of energy art all together.

I personally believe that the Universe is energy that exists on many infinite layers. We all perceive this energy from different perspectives and it is the unique perspective of the individual that is important, not the name or label.

We will never be able to prove conclusively, that the Celts worked with a life-force called Nearth and if this is the same or not the same as Celtic Reiki, because even if we discovered some form of evidence one way or the other, our connection to the more subtle layers of energy is based upon a unique, internal experience that words cannot describe or define.

On some level I know that the experiences I have had with Celtic Reiki are a part of other lives too, Celts, Norse, Ancient Egyptian, Lemurian, and so on. None of us had the words to describe these moments and the labels we ascribe to them do very little to convey the depth of emotion and experience we have shared. However, this bond is the Earth reminding us that we are all one, and beyond that, it is the Universe remembering its true nature.

To embrace this idea of perspective and oneness, I originated a duel philosophy in Celtic Reiki practice, so that the Master can experience the two slightly contracting experiences of working with Reiki in the Shinto ethos and Nearth in the modern Celtic perspective. Therefore, whenever you work with any aspect of Celtic Reiki from realms, to techniques, to essences, etc.

You can choose to work from a Reiki viewpoint, or the Nearth. To differentiate between the tradition 'Neart' and this form of energy art, I have chosen the less common 'Nearth' to symbolise the perspective Celtic Reiki Master's use (both spellings have the same pronunciation of 'Nurt').

Each Master will have a preference based on their own view, attitudes and beliefs, though I do sincerely hope that you will adapt your practice and Mastery to encompass both perspectives, as they both have amazing potential when used to meet the needs of the situation.

In terms of practical use, I have defined the difference between these two perspectives (Nearth/Reiki) as follows: Nearth, for me is more akin to a Lost Language, a vibrational form of communication that enables us to reconnect to the Earth, the trees and many other living things. Reiki is a more Universal view of force, the foundation or basic self, reminding us of our true nature and maintaining our alignment with our life-purposes.

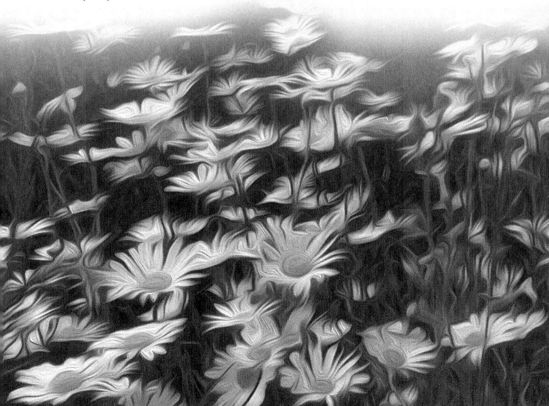

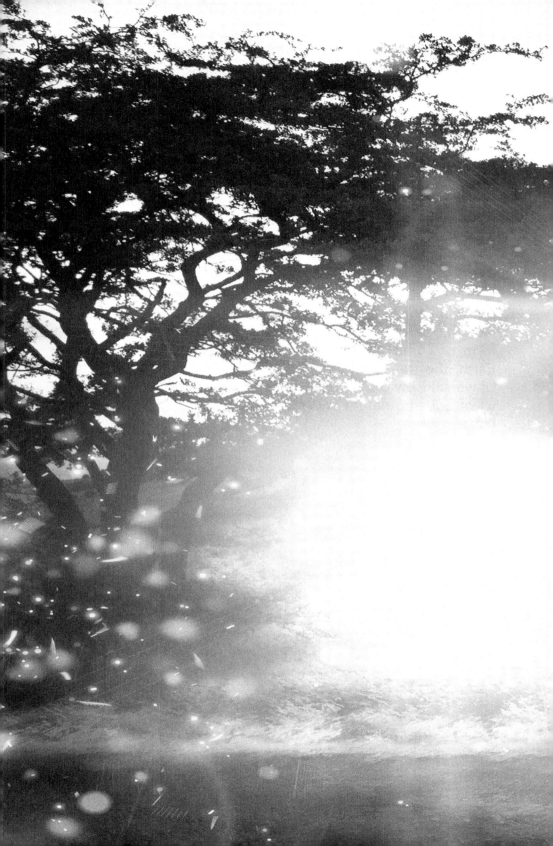

The Lost Language, Rediscovered

Language is often seen as a method of communication, however it is more a means of translation from one thing to another. A computer programming language translates the instructions of a computer user into the binary (zeros and ones) that the computer understands.

Spoken language takes the knowledge of one and transmits it (through writing, verbal means, etc.). Others then filter this transmission in their own perspective, thus translating it to their own interpretation.

When Celtic Reiki first came into being, it was another modality of Reiki practice that could be used for healing or manifestation purposes. As it evolved over time, the therapy was adapted and changed to encompass a more fluid approach to our modern perspective and the history it enveloped. It was not until the very latest layers of Celtic Reiki development that I realised she possessed the sentience of a language; the ability to translate the perspective of the Earth and stars, through trees, living things, minerals, sound and light. The signs were always there, but she had always been defined in the context of a 'therapy' or 'energy art'. When I began to define Celtic Reiki as a lost language, the results expanded beyond anything I, personally, has ever known.

For, as well as retaining all the previous areas of action, Celtic Reiki began to offer ancient wisdom, literally as if spoken across time and space. Thousands of years of knowledge and information, not only in a cultural or human context, but in a multifaceted celebration of life and energy in all its definitions. This lost language translated what had been forgotten into an amazing experience of the present, which presented us with the ability to understand so much unremembered wisdom, but also offered its own key to interpretation; a way of decoding itself so that we may understand the nature of nature.

It was by using the language of Celtic Reiki that we came to realise we are not people relearning old ways and methods, but old ways and methods reimagining ourselves through the gift of consciousness that people offer us.

Hence, the Lost Language of the trees, the Earth, the stars, the ocean, of time and space, is a focal point, a vortex of knowledge that Celtic Reiki Masters connect to so that we can be reborn and experience the wonder of life on Earth and beyond.

In this respect, the language is not only a method that can be used to translate what has been forgotten; it is a way of defining what cannot be defined by words alone.

When a Master defines the world in words, she can only ever define the regions where words exist; however, through the language of Celtic Reiki, no words need exist for there to be a meeting of the physical world and of thought/energy/source, because these elements are translated in ways that the other can comprehend them.

Just as the Shinto philosophy defines Reiki as a bridge between the non-physical Shinki and the physical-world-illusion it creates, we can perceive Celtic Reiki as a bridge (translation) between the stars and the Earth, the past/future and the present, the known and the unknown.

This lost language and our Mastery of it gives us the ability to adapt and translate from a human perspective of ancient wisdom, but as ancient wisdom learning to reclaim its power and potential in the experience of now.

CELTIC REIKI ESSENCES

In many forms of energy art, the concept of energy as a single, all-encompassing force is diluted through the act of definition – 'energies'. This word, and more so the imagery it conjures up, places us in a compartmentalised, 'small' position when working with energy. In my opinion, it deprives us of the holistic nature of Celtic Reiki and offers a foundation that is critically flawed. Imagine referring to a person as 'people' or a tree as a 'forest'. Energy is a totally interconnected entity that is misunderstood by the use of the plural terminology that is so often ascribed to it.

I believe this is one of the absolute foundations of Celtic Reiki Mastery, because it acts as a basis for the realisation that you are not simply mastering Celtic Reiki practice, you are mastering your understanding of energy, force, the Universe and the self; all of which are 'one'.

For, when you divide energy up into sections, you are not only forming very necessary definitions that distinguish one 'entity' from another, you are also creating barriers that make one 'entity' both removed from and different to another. On one hand, this provides contrast, and, on the other, it feeds the illusion of separateness.

Therefore, each Master has the option of determining each situation they encounter, as one where they need distance from the focus of their practice (thus creating definition), or one where they want greater integration (definition between the Master and the focus becomes singular and perspective-orientated).

To reduce the 'compartmentalisation' within Celtic Reiki Mastery, I believe the concept of essences creates a dynamic where energy is viewed with 'oneness', yet differentiation between different experiences of energy can be defined.

Thus, all essences are the same, except for a solitary, but vital parameter: perspective. The essence is the entire Universe, viewed from a unique perspective; for example, the Duir Essence is the Universe as perceived from the perspective of Oak trees. In some circumstances this essence is the view of an individual Oak, in others the perspective of many Oaks, and when typically used, the 'underlying' perspective of the species, Oak. There are also instances, such as Ailim, where the perception of similar species comes together (Fir, Conifer, Spruce, and Pine) and even some essences that offer rather contrasting views, such as in the case of Muin (the Vine and the Bramble).

As you Calibrate to each essence, you are presented with one view of those essences –this is your own, unique perspective of the essences of the particular Orientation. From that point on, you will adapt and change essences according to your own view or perspective.

This may come about through personal choice and, in many instances, through interaction with others. Every treatment you conduct, manifestation routine you work through, or Orientation you present to others, returns an alternative perspective – that of your client or student. As you recognise this new view of Celtic Reiki, so you will shift and transform your own perspective to encompass this additional information.

This is another aspect in the principles of the essence that I feel is very special; because in other forms of energy art, 'types' or 'flavours' of energy remain the same and arrive with their own, predetermined range of 'right' and 'wrong' methods. You may experience a 'type' of Reiki one way, but if this is not how it is 'supposed' to be felt then you are 'wrong' in the way you sense the energy.

With essences there is no correct way of sensing or feedback that is erroneous – there is only your way and my way and both can coexist harmoniously, adding and enriching the other's existence.

ORIENTATION, CORE STATE AND CALIBRATION

The most mysterious and profound cornerstone of any Reiki style is the 'attunement', a sacred process that can be life-changing and transformative in unimaginable ways. Although this somewhat enigmatic process is often quite inconceivable to the Apprentice, its effects are regularly dramatic and awe-inspiring to the extent that many become completely enamoured with the experiences of the attunements.

Originally titled 'empowerments' and what I now call the 'Orientation and Calibration' processes, attunements are an alternative way of teaching people how to work with Reiki and other facets of energy.

Based upon very ancient arts, reported to have been used by mystics for many thousands of years, it is becoming increasingly accepted that the mystery of the attunement process is most likely due to our cultural attitudes than the actual process itself. In fact, the more we understand about the Universe and the way things work beyond our experience of the physical world, the greater the likelihood of attunements being the 'normal' way of things, as opposed to some strange and clandestine practice.

Having had many evolutions over time, the method used in Celtic Reiki training is very different in routine to those used historically. In the Mastery of Celtic Reiki we enter a profound, 'Core State', that removes us from the thoughts and cerebral processes that usually (and constantly) vie for our attention. In this non-reactive state, we can hone and 'Calibrate' our conscious awareness towards a specific outcome or result.

In this instance, the 'Orientation' that your Celtic Reiki Master presents you with.

The best way to describe what is happening, in the Energy Orientation and Calibration process, is to imagine that you are speaking to somebody who had never seen the colour blue – how would you describe this to them in words so that they could understand what you mean? It is virtually impossible!

However, if you could show them a piece of blue-coloured paper, they would instantly know what blue is and they would never forget it. This is the equivalent of an energy Orientation, which displays incredibly vibrant energy that may not have been experienced consciously before. The act of sensing energy (looking at the blue paper and recognising it consciously) is the Calibration part of the process.

The term 'attunement' has long been a term that I am uncomfortable with, because it presupposes that I am 'doing' something 'to' the student. Every so often, I would be confronted by a workshop attendee who explained that they noticed no sensory experience during the attunement.

So I re-imagined the attunement in the form of the 'Energy Lesson', where I taught a lesson in energy for the student to learn. This simple repositioning of the terminology and explanation created a greater degree of success when teaching the approach to recognising Reiki or some other form of subtle energy.

Despite this shifting of description, the Energy Lesson was still not ideal, because it still placed so much emphasis on the teacher. With the attunement, the Master 'did something to the student' and with the Energy Lesson, the Master 'taught something to the student'.

It was this 'one-sidedness' that initiated the creation of the Orientation and Calibration process, we use on Celtic Reiki events and experiences. The Orientation invites the Apprentice to turn their attention to 'this point' (where Celtic Reiki can be sensed) and the Calibration is where the apprentice monitors their sensory data to decipher how they sense 'this point' to the fullest and most all-encompassing range of experience. This, not only balances the process equally between Master and Apprentice, it also assumes that the student will experience something, albeit to different degrees of sensitivity and with a wider variety of sensory feedback.

It is hardly surprising that this methodology has an extremely positive response and greater success than any of its predecessors.

The introduction of the Core State is also incredibly valuable as an initial process that disconnects the Apprentice from external distraction, focuses their attention on the Orientation and strengthens their ability to dilute internal monologue and other thoughts.

By focusing on the pituitary gland (which is regularly associated with spiritual experiences), the Apprentice triggers psycho-chemical processes that act as a catalyst to the powerful and sometimes overwhelming results of the Orientation.

When conscious awareness of Reiki is achieved via some form of attunement, it will never be forgotten and can always be used even if a Practitioner has not practised for many years. It does take a while to integrate fully with the physiological and cerebral systems, so that the various sensory effects and experiences increase with time, becoming stronger certainly over the three weeks after the Orientation. Of course, the more a person consciously practises the techniques and methods of Celtic Reiki, the better they understand it and the more results they will obtain.

Once an Orientation has been 'Calibrated', a range of sensory experiences become available to the apprentice and a period of profound exploration begins and evolves over time. This is the various Celtic Reiki Essences affecting the body and recognition of these effects supports the development of the Mastery skills.

The reason one may experience these changes is due to the conscious focus adjusting to correlate and understand the information it is receiving from the senses that recognise Reiki (and other forms of vibrational energy).

So, until you learn to consciously recognise the subtleties in the Reiki at a direct, vibrational level, your brain translates Reiki as it would the data provided by your regularly used senses (Synaesthesia). Hence the effects seem to involve your sight, hearing, taste, smell and feeling.

Common effects include: brightly coloured flashes of light, shapes and movement in front of the eyes, distortions, such as that caused by looking through heat, strobe effects, high pitched tones/tinnitus, rapid tapping inside the ear, as if a moth is flying about inside, inexplicable smells/perfumes that last only for a moment, peculiar tastes in your mouth, strange feelings of emotion, tingling, especially in the head, hands and feet, heat in hands, feet or head, pins and needles, trembling or spasms, imagery and 'random' thoughts, emotional outbursts, headaches or cold/flu-like symptoms, extremes of heat and cold, magnetic pulling/pushing in hands or body, vibrations/trembling sensations, especially in the spine, and the feeling of being touched or prodded.

These are just some of the sensory experiences you may find after a Celtic Reiki Orientation and Calibration; however, do not be surprised if you have other effects not mentioned here. These are all natural processes and are in no way detrimental to you. They will also ease and gradually disappear once you have integrated/learnt the elements of the Orientation – so do remember to cherish these effects, they are quite extraordinary and create very treasured memories.

My own training in Reiki empowerment and attunements varied in depth and description, yet it fascinated me to such an extent that I became passionate about the development, testing and application of different forms of teaching/learning experience involved with subtle energy and vibrational work. Over the years, this has evolved not only to spiritual endeavours, but also with regards to subjects as diverse as linguistics and social dynamics.

With an expansion into new ways of teaching concepts and ideas, I have pioneered and experienced hundreds of Orientation styles, in addition to the ability to train others in altered states of awareness and advanced ability, simply by talking to them.

I have devised new ways of 'broadcasting' Orientations at a distance, Self-Calibration to Reiki practices (et al), time-distorted and ongoing forms of Calibration where a person will attune upon activating some event (these are known as Click-Tracks or Triggers), and even Orientation and Calibration through reading text.

It is not only the style of Orientation that is important to keep in mind; it is also the nature of what is Calibrated to. When I learnt Usui Reiki I was taught how to change the 'flavour' of Reiki for the purposes of physical or emotional treatment, for example. I was also taught how to connect to Reiki in different ways, for treatment across a distance or at different points in time, or to conduct Master practices such as attunements.

In Celtic Reiki, the traditions continue with the Orientation of essences (perspectives of Ki), the Orientation of shape (the action and results of Ki) and the Orientation to Energyscape or Ki-scape methods, which are complex dynamics of Ki/energy that conduct a series of defined results, based upon different criteria, etc.

So, not only can you learn different essences, you can shape these to achieve different results and even build shapes and essences into a set of defined 'instructions' to create a multitude of effects.

The major shift in ethos in the Orientation process is that it is not the 'type' of energy that one adjusts; it is the perspective of the energy that is changed. Therefore, energy is energy—it is the same, regardless of our perception. Yet, as we alter our perception of energy, the results and effects we achieve differ greatly.

This can be somewhat unusual to the Apprentice because it 'feels' so different, however when you remember that sunlight remains the same, yet appears so different depending on the time of day on Earth, it is easy to understand how our 'position' or perspective in relation to the energy we experience is so different.

Orientations and Calibration exist at every level of Celtic Reiki training and are often the most pleasurable and anticipated aspect of training. It is upon entering the Mastery of Celtic Reiki that these miraculous processes are the most relevant, because it is here that you learn how to conduct Orientations of different styles and how to teach others to Calibrate to them. What was once a profound experience for the Apprentice, becomes a profound ability for the Master.

You will experience various Orientations during your Core State and Calibration sessions. These include the various Celtic and Non-Celtic Tree Essences, the Elemental Essences and the Woodland (Elven) Essences of the Woodland realm. The Standing Stones has Orientations for the Nordic and Crystal Essences, whilst the Mountain Range covers 'methods' of working with Reiki, such as the harvesting of essences and the shaping of energy.

As the Master Orientates his Apprentices to the five

Realms with their many contrasting and complementary essences, and the Mystics with their individual shaping abilities, a vast collection of styles becomes available for Calibration. This rich and complex tapestry offers a diverse and simply extraordinary series of experiences to be had, not only at the time of Calibration, but for weeks, months, and years to come.

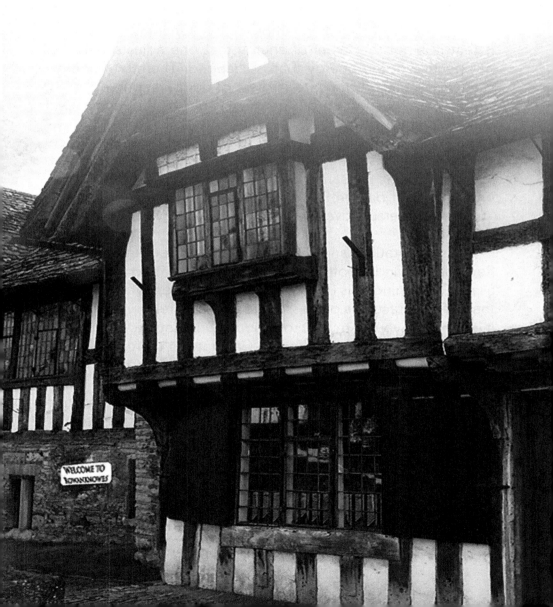

The Five Realms of Celtic Reiki

There are five Celtic Reiki realms for the Adventurer to explore and the Master to command. Each realm encompasses a different range of practice, with its own essences, tools, techniques, and methods. The realms can be seen as categories of Mastery, with each concentrating on a specific aspect of practice.

The Five Realms are:

- The Woodland Realm
- The Standing Stones
- The Celestial Realm
- The Mountain Range
- The Furthest Ocean

Some realms differ only in the type of essence they envelop, whilst others contrast greatly through purpose or aim. For example, the Woodland Realm and Standing Stones are both Essence orientated, with the former containing the Celtic Tree Essences, Elemental Essences, etc. and the later involving the Norse Essences, Crystal Essences, and so on. Then there is the Furthest Ocean that focuses on psychic, intuitive and spiritual abilities, as opposed to essences.

The Realms came about as a way of better managing the vast array of elements to Celtic Reiki, creating classes of essences, techniques and tools that are specific to individual realms and extrapolating methods into their own realm. This maintains a level of autonomy to each realm, yet enables the Master to move between different realms of practice, or even combine them if they wish.

This means, for instance, that if a Master wishes to focus on the Tree-based, Celtic Spirituality of Celtic Reiki they can spend most of their time in the Woodland Realm, alternatively, if they are drawn to crystals and the Norse influences, they can focus their efforts here.

The realms also lean towards different activities or branches of practice; so a healer is likely to spend more time in the Woodland and Celestial Realms, a manifestation-orientated Practitioner would often work in the Standing Stones, whilst a Harvester and Shaper would ascend the Mountain Range, and a Psychic Medium would swim the Furthest Ocean.

With so many different layers to Mastery, it is important that parameters are in place to offer structure and continuity, throughout the diversity that is available to you.

Many Celtic Reiki Masters, who favour one realm, may also find that as their perspective evolves over time, they become interested in the other realms and so, broaden their practice accordingly. Masters can therefore identify themselves generically as a 'Realm Master' or specialise as: a Woodland, Stone, Celestial, Mountain, or Oceanic Master. (We shall cover Mystics in the next section, however these identities can be translated to any Mystic, for example, the Oceanic Warrior or Stone Alchemist, etc.)

The way each realm affects our Mastery is through the dynamic it creates in practice. Dynamics create various effects in the same way that sound is different in air and water, or light is changed by angle. To understand this, think about putting your head into a box and shouting, as compared to shouting on a mountain summit, or how different sunlight appears at midday and at twilight.

The Woodland Realm dynamics are what I would describe as a dance of light and leaf – they exist where the solid world and the energetic Universe meet. These dynamics are powerful and physical, yet light and expansive.

The Standing Stone dynamics are of the Earth and thus better suited to situations where one wants to bring things to ground or contract into the psychical (hence their excellent manifestation abilities). If the Woodland dynamics dance and fizz, the Stone dynamics are always moving into the physical world.

There is a contrasting or even conflicting range of

dynamics in the Celestial Realm. These dynamics travel from the world of solid things, into the ethereal. They are expansive, moving into the unknown, eternal, or infinite. Whenever you work with these dynamics, you are invited to evolve, step forward and move into spiritual layers of greater expansion.

At either end of the Mountain Range, the dynamics form fluid, shaping, moulding and malleable perspectives of energy, so there we discover definition and shape, as well as change and transformation. This realm is the crucible of metamorphosis from one thing into another, but also the fixing of things through definition and complex parameters.

The final set of dynamics exists at a greater layer of contraction than the others. So, the results of the Furthest Ocean are more physical and less expanded than other realm dynamics, but they have a greater influence on the physical world. These are closer to thought than spirit, more in tune with the dynamics of time and space, rather than those of eternity and infinity.

To understand the Celtic Reiki Realms more clearly, let us look at each in turn in greater detail. You can also use the online content from your online Sacred Space to venture further into the heartland of each.

THE WOODLAND REALM

The enchantment of an old, mystical forest is home to more than trees and other plants. The watchful eyes of elf and deva look out at those who walk the old forest paths and sit in ancient clearings to rest, to eat, and to bathe in the sunlight before venturing onwards, under the shade of the canopy.

The Woodland Realm not only embraces the trees, it is of the place between the trees, as if the realm is the space all around us. Within the Woodland Realm, you will encounter the Celtic Reiki Tree Essences, both Celtic and Non-Celtic varieties, the Woodland or Elven Essences and the Elemental Essences that lead you to other realms in your Celtic Reiki Mastery. Therefore, the experienced Celtic Reiki Master will align with the Woodland Realm initially, although a natural alignment will occur when you use any essence of this particular realm.

There are similarities between the Woodland Realm and

both the Standing Stones and the Celestial Realm, because in many ways, the woodland is the meeting point of sky and Earth.

Trees are of the Earth and spend their lives in the ground, yet they strive to reach the light and dance in the sun's glorious rays. It is this synthesis that all plants possess, which enables us to live in the physical world. Without air to breathe and the basic foods that create a foundation for the food-chain, there would be no life on Earth.

So, in the Woodland Realm we connect to the dynamic of expansion, as with the Celestial Realm, yet remain grounded at all times, akin to the Standing Stones dynamic. The result is a dance of light and solid matter that exists at the fundamental levels of the Universe and on many other layers of existence.

The Tree Essences of Celtic Reiki are of the woodland or forest, each essence representing the perspective of a tree or shrub. These interact with each other, with the main goal of growing and developing, both individually and as part of a group.

By Calibrating their perspective to the Woodland Realm, the Master creates an outcome that behaves as a forest behaves; a complex system of life, growth, expansion and connection to the Earth. This realm represents a sacred, peaceful and enchanted place where one can heal, learn, explore, discover, create, relax, and find spiritual awakening.

The woodland envelops all four elements, through the spatial perspective of the realm: a tree grows in the Earth, drinks water, processes the air, and feeds on sunlight (fire). As these are all done in space and time, the main concept of the Woodland Realm is of a spatial dynamic through which we create a range of powerful results with the trees, woodland dwellers and elements.

The Elemental Essences of the Woodland Realm have rather unique qualities, because they connect us to the other realms. The Pridd Essence (Earth) opens a gateway to the Standing Stones, Annal (Air) connects us to the Celestial Realm, whilst Tan (Fire) is a portal to the Mountain Range and finally Dwr (Water) is our link to the Furthest Ocean.

When we use these essences, they form an automatic connection to the other realms. Once this occurs we can choose to make the transition to the individual realms and continue our Celtic Reiki work from there, or to stay in the Woodland Realm and use the other aspects of the Elemental Essence we are Calibrated to.

THE STANDING STONES

This realm envelops the crystal and mineral essences, as well as drawing from Norse culture and theology; a counterpart to that of the Celts. The Runic symbolism that is associated with these essences mirrors the Ogham and thus, offers a symmetrical beauty to the tree and crystal essence use.

The Standing Stones are of the Earth, though through the contractive dynamics they create, a connection to the Celestial Realm and to the air is made. As the Essences of this realm bring situations and circumstance into the physical they travel from the ethereal of the Celestial Realm.

One way of looking at this, is that even though crystal and mineral are the Earth, the base minerals come from the stars. Linked through physical history to what is beyond the Earth, the stones are akin to the trees, inasmuch as there is a connection between the Earth and sky, albeit very different in actual dynamic.

Whilst there are many connections and similarities between the tree and the stone, their consciousness of each is very different; the stone exists upon distant, intangible layers of perception, way beyond the usual perception of people. Crystals display the three requirements to be classed as 'living'; they grow, they reproduce and they communicate, for if a crystal is struck, other crystals in the vicinity will display a change in vibration also.

Research shows that this same effect can be measured in crystals that are situated in completely different parts of the world.

These qualities offer the Celtic Reiki Master a detailed understanding of the Earth at deep levels of perception. The wisdom of the trees spans lifetimes of hundreds, even thousands of years. Yet, the stones represent millions of years of life, which extends to billions in some essences and through the foundations of every Nordic Stone Essence.

In many ways these essences represent the life of the

Earth. Therefore, if the trees represent the ever-changing, fleeting moment of experience; stone essences provide a deep-rooted grounding that transcends time. There are still adaptations, but these are so distended over time, as to be indiscernible without drastic alterations in perception.

The essences of the Standing Stones are excellent when used in manifestation techniques and treatments. They also show remarkable power in healing and the pursuit of knowledge (both of which are forms of manifestation too: the manifestation of health and of wisdom).

The bringing of things, states of being, situations, and so on, from the ethereal into the 'real' world is a contractive process that occurs through the interaction of energy. However, it is interesting to note that whilst the stones are 'of the past', their essences are 'of the now', having the effect of contraction (turning future into past, or energy into solid).

Therefore every essence of the Standing Stones exists in the moment it is used (though it exists beyond space and time). The results it has affect space and time, thus creating results that are susceptible to age.

A wonderful analogy of this is the Volcano that takes the fluid potential of the Earth that cannot be measured in isolated 'chunks' and creates new rock or minerals, yet as soon as these are formed, they begin to age. The rock/mineral can be dated through definition, but not through transition of its foundation energy. Hence, the results of the Standing Stone essence are measurable in the physical world, but remain infinite in energy terms.

THE CELESTIAL REALM

The dynamic of the Celestial Realm is of expansion into the unknown, the future, the greater self and transcendence of the physical, for it exists beyond the movements of three-dimensional perception. This can be confusing for the new Adventurer, because in the physical world, we are so used to paths and the 'normal' way of things.

When the Adventurer sets out into the forest, she knows that the path she walks has been walked by many others, yet when she looks down to her feet, she sees that she is creating the path as she goes. In the Celestial Realm, there are no paths or linear journeys.

Here, the Adventurer moves beyond the physical world and comes to know the layers of perception, which exist beyond human comprehension. The Celestial Realm is truly alien in its very fabric, not only because it is not of the Earth, but it is not of regular human perception.

The Celestial Realm is of the element of Air, and symbolises this in many ways; from the concept of ascendance, to being 'up in the air'. The motion of air is also encapsulated in this realm, from the stillness of a summer's day to the howling wind, the slow, indiscernible moment of air to the hurricane.

The Stellar Essences (planets, stars and constellations) are equated with the Celestial, which also represents the connection to otherworldly places, far off locations and the 'Stargate Essence'.

When we compare this realm to that of the Woodland and our tree essences, we gain a greater insight in the results that the Celestial dynamics produce. For trees and humans alike, the Earth is our home and all that we have ever known in physical terms.

When people harvest or connect to tree essences, we are so alike in many ways It is because of these shared connections that it feels very natural. There are so many truly incomprehensible aspects to the Celestial Realm that it becomes very apparent when a perspective is human or alien.

We each have our own perspective of 'The Plough' constellation, though when you experience this essence from a truly alien perspective, it changes you at a fundamental level. You never quite see the world in the same way again and the experience can really help you to appreciate the precious nature of life and the awe-inspiring beauty around us in ways that are unlike the usual perspective.

It is an interesting element of this Realm that the civilisations most connected with the expansion of our awareness as a species of the planets and stars were the Greeks and Romans, but Ancient Egyptians were also fascinated by the night sky and its mysteries. The system of Celtic Reiki encompasses all of these perspectives (over 10,000 years of philosophy), having become the energy art of indigenous culture, the natural world and what lies beyond the world.

This is illustrated as the exploration of our ancestry extends into the furthest reaches of our past, to a point where history and mythology blur into strange places that seem only to exist in the innermost reaches of our core perception; the prehistoric, lost civilisations of the world.

When the Adventurer explores the Standing Stones, he begins from the perspective of expanded awareness and contracts into the physical world, thus manifesting certain outcomes. Yet, when he journeys through the Celestial Realm, his contracted perspective is expanded into the unknown.

Here knowledge, experience and perception are all important and have a major impact on what the Adventurer chooses to manifest and explore in the future. Consequently, the Celestial is the emblem of future adventures and future-selves, compared to the historical, past emphasis of the Standing Stones. Nonetheless, the essences of the Celestial Realm exist in the present moment, as do all essences and perspectives of energy.

The Mountain Range

There are many lost civilisations that existed long before the written word came about. There remain remnants of some of these societies and cultures, such as the Ancient Egyptians, Mayans, and Aztecs, however many are said to be completely lost, except in some deep inner-knowing that many share. Two infamous examples of these civilisations are the Lost Cities of Atlantis and Lemuria.

In Celtic Reiki philosophy, we work with both Lemuria and Atlantis; however we focus more on the core dynamics of these concepts as opposed to seeing them as actual places. Atlantis is renowned for its technological achievement, with a profound grasp of geometry and form.

A physically-based society, physicality, shape and geometry are the elements that play an important part of the Mountain Range dynamic. Conversely, Lemuria is believed to be ethereal in nature, with a greater understanding of the unique perspective every individual possesses and how this affects a community or group.

The Lemurians are often said to be energy beings, or

not of physical form, in this place, between the solid world and the realm of energy, they created form through definition and parameterisation.

This wonderfully intricate, yet beautifully simple relationship between the Lemurian and Atlantean perspectives is at the heart of the Mountain Range philosophy and indeed the core principles of Celtic Reiki.

Energy is intangible and amorphous in its Universal state, though, as soon as it is defined through the perspective of an individual it can be shifted and moulded in the physical world. The definitions offered by perspective leads to the Atlantean dynamic of shaping and change, through a powerful layering of parameters that form energy of a simple action and reaction, or of complex diversity and continuity.

As the Adventurer enters the Mountain Range, she gazes across a panorama that extends from the high mountains at the north of the range, to the volcanoes of the south. The peaks of the northern mountains are so massive that the entire realm can be seen from the highest of these.

This area of the Mountain Range represents the observer, the viewpoint and the perspective from which all else is perceived and defined. The philosophy of the northern peaks is one of the uniqueness that every observer has through their own senses and interpretation.

The fiery southern volcanoes emulate the concept of adaptation, moulding and shaping of the world. Just as everything is cleansed and reborn through fire, so our perception can also be adapted through the shaping of energy, thought and connection. This Atlantean view of geometric shaping, combined with the perspective orientation of the Lemurian view provide Masters with an adaptability in their art unlike anything else available in our field.

One of the very first pieces of knowledge the Adventurer gleans as she traverses the peaks of the Mountain Range is the relationship between the observer and the observed: how one body can be changed through the act of being observed and how this same body then changes the observer.

The Adventurer recognises the many essences of the different realms, they also understand each from an infinite array of perspectives and reshape essences into forms as simple as a line, or as complex as the multi-faceted thought patterns of the genius mind.

It is in the Mountain Range Realm where harvesting and definition of the essences takes place, as the Celtic Reiki Master orientates to the perspective of trees, stones, the stars and the Earth. Once orientated, they adapt the parameters for their intents and create their own Mastery of Celtic Reiki, with personal essences and a vast array of unique tools that are personally-defined.

THE FURTHEST OCEAN

As the Adventurer dives into the Furthest Ocean and its endless depths of emotion, perception and cerebral creation, they are immersed in the element of water and all its mystery. The oceanic realm is very different to that of the land; it holds secrets and enigma beyond imagination and yet, the ocean is not the external place we believe it to be: it represents the internal world and the hidden knowledge we all possess at our very foundation.

The relationship between the Celestial Realm and the Standing Stones is like two equal and opposing forces that create balance and harmony. Each pushes against the other to form a central point of stability and strength through (in the case of these two realms) contraction and expansion into each other. The Furthest Ocean and Mountain Range share this same relationship of opposition and balance, yet here we also see unity and similarity.

Both the water and the fire realms consist of the act of definition. Yet, the Mountain Range enables us to take the intangible and to define it into the physical world.

The Furthest Ocean is the art of redefinition; observing that which is stagnant or dogmatised through old, overused, or overly-simplified definition and creating new parameters that realign with the intangible and infinite.

An example of this is how Usui Reiki practice seemed so new and revolutionary when I first studied the philosophy and attunement. Within the space of four to five years, however, it became a rigid, conflicted practice, with much internal contention and back-biting.

My personal solution to this was to work through the

Oceanic dynamic to redefine Reiki practice into something that is far more complex and challenging to master, yet much more fluid, individual, and relevant to contemporary society. I have continued this process with Celtic Reiki, reworking, adapting and reimagining the system every few years.

In practical, everyday terms, the psychic abilities offered through the Furthest Ocean grant the adventurer (and other Mystics) access to intuition when treating, the ability of divination in Celtic Reiki readings and the empathy of higher cerebral abilities that give the impression of telepathy and a deep knowing of others' needs.

Connection to ancient wisdom and the intelligences that exist beyond our time and space are gained by swimming in the ocean, yet the emphasis is always on redefinition and a return to the intangible so that we may be inspired to journey onwards into the unknown depths.

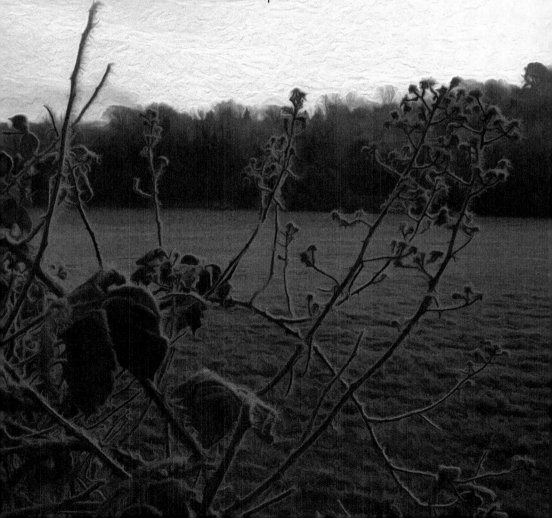

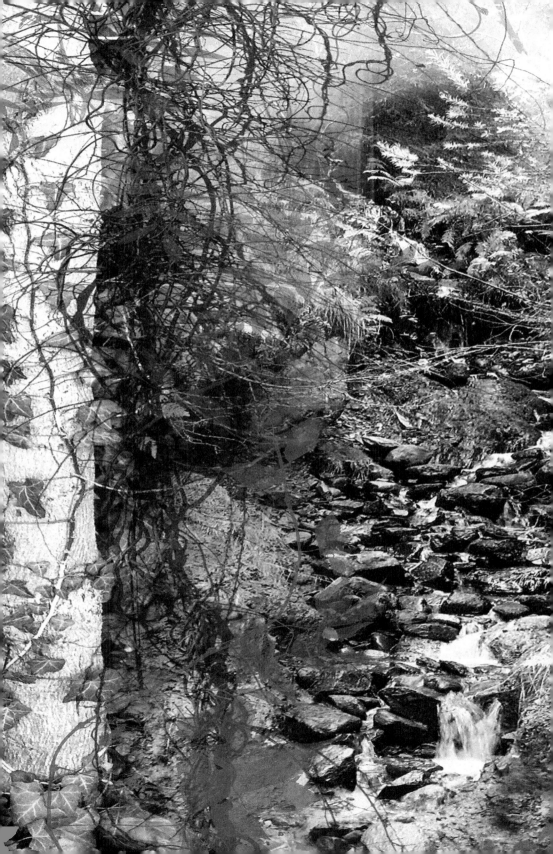

THE FIVE MYSTICS OF CELTIC REIKI

A revolutionary way of working with Celtic Reiki is with the concept of the Mystics. These symbolic beings represent the perspective that a practice or treatment is conducted from. As you work with the various essences, techniques, styles, and so on, you alter the perspective of the treatment by working in 'avatar' state to connect to the individual Mystics. There are in fact two ways of viewing this process and you can choose which one you prefer to work with. The first approach is that you act as an avatar for the different Mystic personas and the alternative is that the Mystic is an avatar that you step into. Either way, there is not actually any 'stepping' or 'becoming', it is merely a shift of viewpoint that takes place.

Imagine several people standing in a valley, with some atop a high crest and others down in the valley itself. Some look down and focus on the beauty of the place, whilst others would be weighing up its potential value on the land market. There are those that would look up and see a challenge and some who feel the climb is too much like hard work! Every perspective is not only different in physical location, but also contrasting in psychological perspective. The Mystics act in a similar way to alter your perspective of a treatment or practice.

The five Mystics of Celtic Reiki will help you, in avatar state, to alter the results you achieve, through the different perspectives. These five Mystics are:

- The Alchemist
- The Wise One
- The Adventurer
- The Warrior
- The Master

Each Mystic has an individual and unique way of perceiving the world, the situation you're treating and the focus of the treatment, be it a client, a dynamic or you.

The Wise One will conduct any practice with the intention of gaining knowledge, expanding the consciousness, and improving ability, whereas the Alchemist will be looking to attain better results and achieve more through combination and a blending of different techniques, essences, etc.

The Adventurer that you Calibrated to in the initial Celtic Reiki Orientation is the very first Mystic an apprentice encounters. The Adventurer is an excellent Mystic to explore the realms of Celtic Reiki and get a deep understanding for the different realms, Lores, essences, and so on.

When you work with the Adventurer in avatar state, you become curious and questioning, yet confident in your ability to find answers and walk onwards on the epic journey of exploration that is Celtic Reiki…

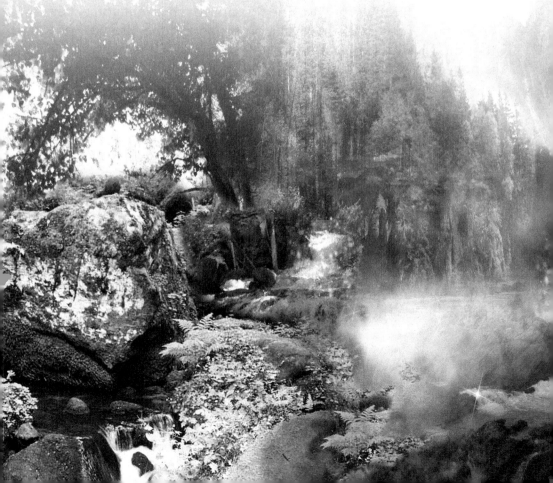

THE ADVENTURER

As the Adventurer you are an explorer, a student, and a discoverer of uncharted territory. The purpose of enveloping this avatar is to learn more about an essence, technique realm or practice in the Celtic Reiki Mastery. This Mystic helps you, not only to learn Celtic Reiki practice, but also to explore and discover new layers of wonder in the advancement of your development practices and mastery.

Treatments, essences, etc. are automatically experienced at a deeper level of sensory perception whenever you embody the Adventurer Mystic. There is an increased awareness of how you are affected by any practice, accompanied by a pushing outwards of your current boundaries to glean 'more' from Celtic Reiki – more experience, more sensation, more awareness, more knowledge, and so on.

Whereas the Warrior is simply confident about their overall ability, the Adventurer is bold, with amazing self-esteem and total confidence in the abilities they can achieve. To the Adventurer, what some may call 'mistakes' are seen as opportunities.

When a wrong-turn is taken, the Adventurer will learn as much as they can, so as to create change in the future and to develop a wise understanding of how the right, future path for each situation can be intuitively discovered.

THE WARRIOR

The Warrior Mystic has a determination that is unlike any other. They know that a person can do anything they set their mind to, providing they are willing to do what it takes to succeed. When you calibrate to the Warrior Mystic during the Practitionership of your adventure, you will be able to work through avatar state to have confidence in your ability, methodology and knowledge.

Whereas the Adventurer explores and discovers, the Warrior displays the courage to explore beyond the comfort zone, to innovate and have faith in what is discovered. The Warrior Mystic also asserts the results they achieve, so when a client is resistant, because of scepticism or limiting belief, the Warrior will guide the client to transcend what is keeping them from expanding and assist in their personal growth.

No Celtic Reiki Master can make their client well, or manifest a goal on their client's behalf – for it is our job to act simply as a catalyst to the process.

The client (or focus) must take on the responsibility for their own ability to heal, manifest, etc. for any practice to work, however, imagine a scenario where a car mechanic and a doctor give you a diagnosis for a headache; whose opinion would you trust and more importantly, who do you feel is more likely to help ease the headaches? This is the role of the Warrior, because by believing in yourself, you inspire others to believe in themselves also.

The Warrior is also an excellent Mystic to work with, in avatar state, when conducting Celtic Reiki readings, because they will increase the strength of the reading and connect at a greater sensory level to the information.

In turn this offers heightened clarity in visualisation and interpretation of the readings. Furthermore, the Warrior is the Mystic of psychic perception and encounters of the paranormal/ otherworldly when working in a Celtic Reiki context.

THE WISE ONE

When you work through avatar state to connect with the wisdom of the Wise One you become a healer and a keeper of secrets. As you progress from the student and explorer phase of your Celtic Reiki adventure, the Practitioner enters a layer of experience that requires compassion, unconditional care and the ability to transcend one's own boundaries. Even in the Mastery of Celtic Reiki, the Wise One Mystic is revisited on a regular basis.

Treatments and practices that are conducted from the perspective of the Wise One take on a deep-acting quality that is centred on healing of past trauma and current challenges. The healer is also the contemplative; a profound being that gleans wisdom from every experience and learns from the situations they encounter.

As you work with the Wise One, particularly with treatments, you immerse yourself in the processes of the treatment and learn from them for future use. Knowledge and experience simply 'stick' with greater adhesion to the memory of this Mystic.

An integral part of the third Orientation, along with the Alchemist Mystic, the Wise One creates an ongoing and adaptive avatar that will be a steady companion on your Celtic Reiki path. If the Adventurer is seen as expansion and the Warrior is strengthening; the Wise One would be integration to create an all-encompassing, balanced, and evolving perspective.

In visual terms we could imagine the Alchemist to be the eyes focusing in on a distant object, to clarify it, the Wise One is an acknowledgment of the peripheral vision to absorb as much of a scene as possible.

THE ALCHEMIST

The Alchemist favours the manifestation or creation of dreams in the physical world, when conjuring something new from two or more elements. The Magician and Spell Caster of the Celtic Reiki Realms, the Alchemist Mystic helps the Practitioner or Master bring what is wished for into reality.

The attainment of goals is a process that transcends mere fancy – it requires planning and regular assertion, yet the power of the Alchemist inspires results that bring what is potential into reality.

Imagine wanting something so much (or not wanting it) that you think about that thing most of the time. Eventually, according to the magnetic laws of the Universe, you will bring that 'thing' towards you.

Yet the mere dreaming and visualisation of that end result may create a meandering effect where the goal takes time to manifest or a dual-effect where ambiguous results are created. The focused, quantified results of the Alchemist create huge momentum and assist in the clarification surrounding manifestation and the goals a person requires.

Additionally, the Alchemist is excellent when used at the Master degree to harvest and create essences. Now, whilst the Warrior is often a better choice when working on the testing of essences, the Alchemist will enhance the definition of essences, honing in on results and effects.

In many ways, Celtic Reiki essences rely a great deal on the parameters set by each individual Master, and this Mystic not only helps create an arena for clear definition, but also hones every aspect of an essence into easily definable characteristics.

THE MASTER

We shall explore the enigmatic nature of the Master Mystic in the final book of your Home Experience, for there is much to learn between then and now. The role of the Master Mystic is primarily as a Mentor and Teacher, whose connection to Celtic Reiki overflows with integrity and the ability to instil that connection in others. The Master creates circumstances that are excellent for training others and the creation of learning environments.

The role of the Master Mystic has a far broader range of influence than simply teaching, as they nurture an outlook of compassion and kindness, as well as strength of mind and spirit. A leader and guide to those who seek expansion and growth, the Master is connected to many secrets and sacred knowledge that can be accessed and imparted to inspire others with grace and power.

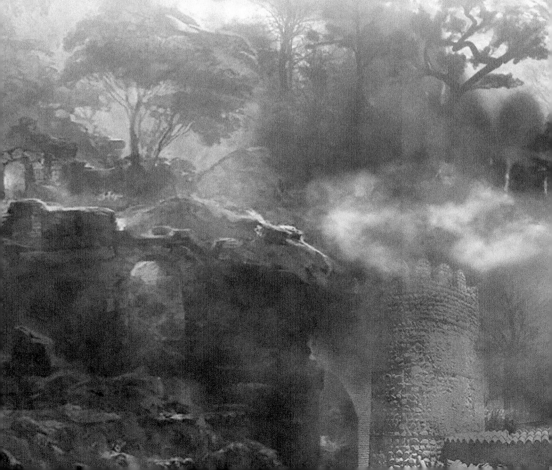

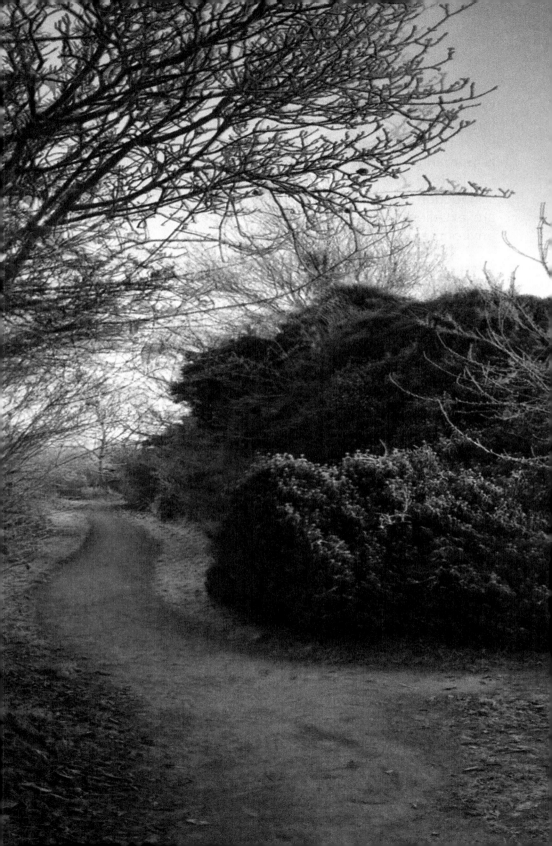

THE FIVE LORES OF CELTIC REIKI

Lore is the *way of things*; like the natural flow of water in a stream, or how clouds move across the sky on a breezy day. Whereas *laws* are how something must be according to the perspective and parameters of a particular focus, lore changes from moment to moment, yet remains timeless in relevance and continuity.

The five Lores of Celtic Reiki are guidelines, methodologies or ways of doing specific activities that can be viewed as a support framework for Celtic Reiki practice. With the potential for such scope in method and adaptability, there needs to be some form of definition that states *this is Celtic Reiki and that is not*.

The five main Celtic Reiki Lores present a basic framework for learning, practice and teaching that explain some inherent methods and philosophies of Celtic Reiki methodology. To act within the definition of the Lores gives Masters and other users of the Celtic Reiki system peace of mind that they are offering their clients treatments, etc. with a spirit or viewpoint that is integrally *Celtic Reiki*, even though they have adapted and evolved the system. The Lores are not exclusive, but they do offer some precepts into the appropriateness of a particular way of acting.

One final important area of this debate is how, in any practice that can be adapted so widely, it is vital to maintain the attitude of choice and flexibility, as opposed to dogma and rigidity. For instance, I love the colour yellow, however I do not believe yellow is the *best* colour or indeed the *only* colour.

A habit has formed in Reiki practices (as with many other practices) of taking the attitude of *my way is the right way*. We create paths through the decisions we make and the actions we take—these paths are choices, not absolute 'law'. I would say that many people have a favourite colour and that it is good to eat food, however, beyond that it all boils down to personal preference.

No matter how Celtic Reiki is adapted or changed, I ask that each Celtic Reiki Master (and Masters of all Reiki methods) develop an attitude of differentiating personal choice from absolute law. The realisation that any adaptation—or even original concept—is based on a particular perspective that can change and evolve, persuades us to be clear about what is my way and how this can help you find your way, but will never be your way.

When we examine the Lores, we see that Celtic Reiki embodies TreeLore, whilst Usui Reiki is often fixed in EarthLore and both have elements of EnergyLore and DarkLore.

In recent years Usui Reiki has been focused on *getting back to the way it was originally done* and has thus become more focused on EnergyLore, whereas I feel the original system, created by Usui, had a greater emphasis on DarkLore. I believe Celtic Reiki is most effective when used with a synchronisation of all five Lores—with a central Lore as the focus and the other four, concurrently and consistently positioned in the periphery of conscious awareness.

EARTHLORE

EarthLore is the definition of our sensory and emotional experience of the Earth, as part of ourselves. Earthlore touches our conscious experience of all things, including spirituality and thought, which means that whilst our focus may lie with things beyond the physical world, we have a tendency to filter those things through the perception of our Earthly experience.

Reiki as a force is part of CosmicLore, however our intellectual perception of Reiki and its ability to power treatments, manifestation, etc. is of the EarthLore. In other words, Reiki undefined is CosmicLore, the act of definition would be TreeLore and the experience of Reiki within the context of that definition is EarthLore.

EarthLore represents the world and everything that is part of the world – it is the Earth and therefore it is the physical body. The body you believe yourself to be is of the Earth and whilst there is more that exists beyond the physical world, our skill at placing parameters on the world around us and for it to parameterise us in return creates the world and is the core theme of EarthLore.

Therefore, EarthLore covers the methods and systems, the tools and techniques, and the principles and philosophies of Celtic Reiki. For example, the creation (in the sense of definition and application) of a Celtic Reiki Essence is EarthLore, as are the treatment methods used and the discernible results. The experience of an essence during treatment is not of EarthLore (this is TreeLore).

When it comes to your individual Mastery of Celtic Reiki, EarthLore is your arena of creation, because although much EarthLore is presented to you through your training, we each discover and define our own EarthLore along the way.

So, for example, a particular essence may come with its own prescriptive definition (range of treatment suggestions), you may find that you have completely different results. It is these results that define the EarthLore of your practice, along with the techniques, tools, and other methodologies you personally apply to your Mastery.

CosmicLore

CosmicLore is beyond our world, for it is of the stars; the intangible; the unknowable. When we look up at the night sky, we do not look through space, we look back through time, because we are not sensing what is, but what was.

Always one step behind, our senses and Earthly experience is always of what was and never of what is. 'What is', is of the CosmicLore—the unknown and the undefined. As soon as you create parameters through TreeLore, so that CosmicLore can be grasped by the conscious mind, it is no longer of CosmicLore, but of EarthLore.

Imagine that you visited a beautiful landscape ten years ago and whilst you were there, you took a photograph of the landscape. Before and after your visit, the landscape would be CosmicLore—unknown and outside of usual physical perception.

During your visit and picture-taking, the landscape (and your observation of it) is TreeLore, and now, ten years later, as you gaze at the photograph, it is EarthLore, along with your memories of the landscape. You cannot say, using the usual sensory abilities, what the landscape would be at this exact moment, but you can say what it 'was' like to you ten years ago and what that memory means to you know.

CosmicLore is potential and also truth – the paradox is that as soon as we perceive it, it is no longer either and yet is remains both! Space and Time are both EarthLore, so when we define with those EarthLore parameters, we create more of the same, however the foundations (potential and truth) still exist in CosmicLore; they are simply negated in EarthLore, because of our integral grounding in the physical, defined world.

ENERGYLORE

EnergyLore is best described as what we perceive as the external existence, becoming the internal experience, or in more basic terms; the outside world flowing into you.

Within the parameters of EarthLore, the Sun shines energy through space and in time to the Earth, where we experience it spatially and chronologically. The point is that sunlight does not travel anywhere; it simply exists in different states of being. In one state it is of the sun and in another state it is of your experience of the sun.

EnergyLore is therefore a dynamic that is present whenever what is 'outside' becomes what is 'inside'. The Orientation element of attunement to Celtic Reiki is EnergyLore, as is the cerebral and experiential learning of the practice.

When you take what is without and make it what is within, this is the dynamic of EnergyLore in action. This book is EarthLore, the translation of the words in this book into your individual interpretation and the thoughts that stem from that interpretation are EnergyLore.

This very personal and unique experience reaches deep into your perspective, creates change and growth and evolution and then it turns back on itself and becomes DarkLore.

DARKLORE

If CosmicLore is of the Sun, then DarkLore can be compared with the Moon. Cosmologists believe that the Moon was created when the original Earth collided with another planet, known as Thea.

The two planets impacted and converged to form the Earth and the Moon. Thus, when we look at the Moon (and with acknowledgement to the notion that we are all of the Earth), we perceive what was once internal, in the external world – or what was within, without!

The Moon is often viewed as mysterious and representative of what is hidden. DarkLore mirrors this inasmuch as it is our internal experience of everything we encounter, represented in an external form.

What we do, how we act, the words we speak, write, and so on are all of the DarkLore. The Calibration processes of the Celtic Reiki attunement are DarkLore, as is the adaptation, use and teaching of our individualised forms of Celtic Reiki.

Hence, you might conclude that DarkLore is the reverse of EnergyLore, however, is the darkness really the opposite of light or is it the absence of light? Dark and Light have commonly been set up in opposition to each other, yet darkness is not a 'thing' in itself, it is the perceived lack of a *thing*.

The fascinating question that is derived from this philosophy is, does the 'outside world' exist as a thing within itself, or is it actually the perceived lack of a thing within itself?

TREELORE

TreeLore is the strength that binds all other Lores into our experience. There is a place where the observer (DarkLore) is connected to the observed (EnergyLore) and where what is known (EarthLore) meets that, which is unknown (CosmicLore). Take a look at the symbol for infinity (∞), and you will see that the two loops converge at the middle to a single point and no matter how you travel along the path of the infinity, you will always pass this convergence at some point.

Trees are the place where the heavens meet the Earth, or the physical (leaves) meet the ethereal (sunlight). In this place, a frenetic dance occurs; a tango of energy as light and energy as the solid world. Trees, for me, represent this union of contrast; of abundance and lack; of light and dark; inner and outer; heaven and Earth.

TreeLore is therefore the transformation of one dynamic or Lore into another. Trees symbolise birth, death and rebirth, the past, future and the present, as well as what is above, below and in between. They are the transitional point, where one thing can become something else and as such, TreeLore provides us with a system for change and transcendence.

The *plan* or potential for Celtic Reiki exists in CosmicLore, the actual practice (method and philosophy) exists in EarthLore, yet in TreeLore, every person has the ability to make Celtic Reiki a unique celebration of their own perspective. The seemingly paradoxical element of TreeLore is that it remains a constant in Celtic Reiki practice.

If CosmicLore is infinite in potential and EarthLore is infinite in the perspectives from which it defines, DarkLore is the transport mechanism in one direction and EnergyLore moves us in the opposite direction; it is TreeLore that stays at the heart of the infinity. A single point of experience where personal truth is found and all becomes real, if only for a fleeting second of space and time.

TreeLore

In every moment you are anew: the sum of what you were and what you are and what you have the potential to become. When you look at who you want to be, if you understand that person to be you, in the future, then you are not seeing who you will become, but who you were. When you understand this as another perspective, sensed through the senses of this physical form, you realise a potential that is beyond the limitations of the self and the abilities you believe yourself capable of…

THE WISE OAK

The Adventurer arrived at a sunlit sanctuary, deep in the heart of the forest. It was here that an old, wise Oak tree lifted his branches high into the sky, beyond the reach of the other trees. As the figure came forward, the tree regarded the approach with mild curiosity, for it was not often that a traveller came this far into the forest.

"Are you lost?" Asked the wise old Oak.

"No," The Adventurer replied. "I am simply exploring!"

"The explorer who has not lost themselves will never find much of interest!" remarked the Oak, with an inner-chuckle.

"What do you mean?" The Adventurer was puzzled.

"The most profound wisdom is born from confusion and confusion is the dominion of the one who has lost their way. For if you are not lost, how do you expect to find anything that you do not already know?"

"Please explain further!"

The tree continued, "If you know where you are going, then you already have defined what you expect to find. When you lose your way, you are open to being surprised, when you find where you are going!"

"I'm confused!" said the Adventurer.

"Good!" The tree laughed. "That is the very first step on the way to understanding!"

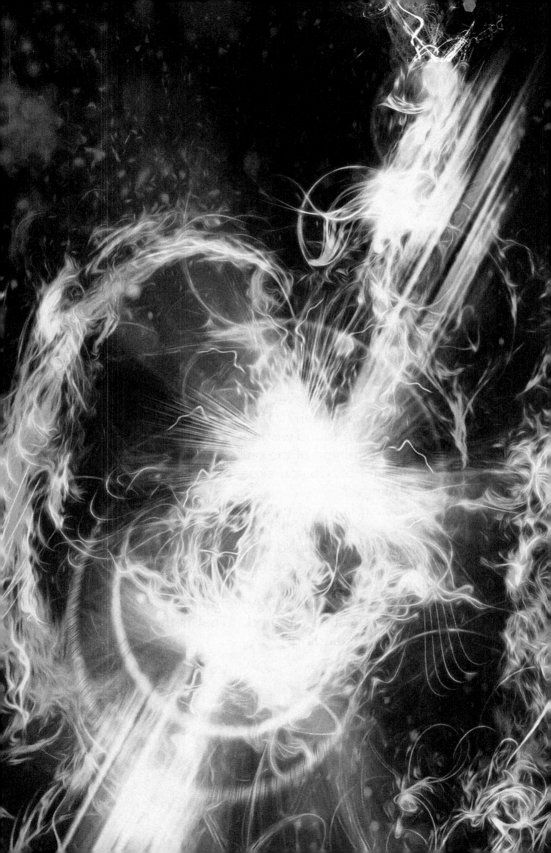

THE FIRST STEPS...

Once you have Calibrated to the initial Orientation of your Home Experience, you will most probably want to experiment with the experiences of working with essences.
You will have already connected to a treatment using essences, however, the experience of shifting your own perception to each essence as an Adventurer will be very different.

During a treatment, the Celtic Reiki Master conducts a set of techniques and uses selected essences in ways that are rather like an Orientation. The most important difference is that you (as the one being treated) do not Calibrate to that Orientation. This can present you with an amazing experience, nonetheless, and the treatment is an excellent introduction into Celtic Reiki.

In many ways, the Celtic Reiki treatment is akin to the basic attunements of Usui Reiki (Degree One) in potency, offering the same level of result.

After Celtic Reiki treatments, people often report a level of sensation and synaesthesia that seem more in line with an 'attunement' in terms of the type of feedback one would expect. The major difference comes with the Calibration, where the Apprentice takes an active role in the discovery of Celtic Reiki from their perspective.

The proactive Calibration will not only provide you with a heightened perception of Reiki (as well as the other facets of Ki) and Nearth, it presents you with your 'own' perspective of these.

This crucial difference ensures that the immediate practices you undertake are an extension or elaboration of this process, rather than learning from the starting point of your Celtic Reiki Master's perspective. The outcomes of this are greater results that are grasped faster, and achieve a deeper integrity of action.

In the following sections, we shall explore some of the tools and techniques that you can use immediately after your first Orientation and Calibration to hone your abilities and help your learning experience for the rest of your training (and beyond!)

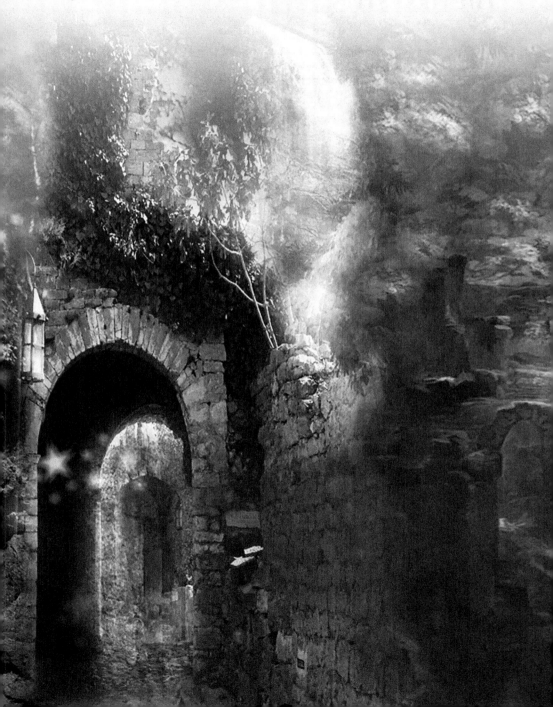

Tree Plans

As Celtic Reiki has evolved over time, it has increased in both intricacy and the ability to deal with the complexity of modern challenges and dis-ease. Some choose to work from their Master perspective with the original simplicity; however, this approach is more in line with the Tribal dynamic and will therefore be ineffective for people who function from the Altruistic Sphere and 'above'.

The Egocentric dynamic is still affected to a great extent by the Tribal perspective, as are all that have progressed beyond the Survival Sphere, though, in the Altruistic dynamic, the Tribal Sphere is actively transcended as too simplistic (or in some cases negative or 'bad').

This is why many people find energy therapies ineffective for their needs – it is not an issue with the therapy, but the perspective from which the therapy is conducted. If a person conducts a treatment from the Sociocentric Sphere, for example, it is likely to have beneficial results for somebody on the Material layer, but not for the Experiential Sphere or above.

When I first started working with Usui Reiki, I found the methods I had been taught worked for some, but not for others. As I expanded all the methods I have pioneered to the Experiential Sphere or beyond, I have increased the level of effectiveness to 100% success with some practices. This is because an activity conducted from the Tribal perspective will only ever work on some layer of a person's conscious perspective (unless they are themselves, in the Tribal perspective). If you work from a perspective at greater expansion from your clients, you are constantly inviting them to expand into the next dynamic.

The Systemic and Experiential Spheres (and beyond) are excellent for the evolutionary processes of humankind, because we can move to other layers and dynamics to achieve the most amazing results. So, in many ways, your first task as an Adventurer is to explore the philosophy of expansion and then find your method of attaining progression beyond the Sociocentric Sphere (if you have not already done so).

The very fact that you are reading these words means that you are very capable of this task. The want of something and the ability to attain it are equal and opposing forces – they push against each other and make the other possible. You enrolled on the Home Experience, because your current ability to successfully complete the programme gave you the force necessary to get this far. To illustrate this, imagine pushing against a sturdy brick wall and then imagine pushing against thin air. Which example offers you the best chance of staying upright?

When I conducted the treatment on the Lone Tree that initiated my own Celtic Reiki adventure, I knew instantly that my first attempts at treating the standing section of the tree and the fallen piece separately, were to no avail: there was no 'resistance'.

Yet, as soon as I altered my approach to connect the two parts of the tree, I knew it was working, because I experienced the force—a force that can only be present if there is something for it to push against. If you are unable to achieve something, you would never want that thing, because there is nothing for the 'want' to 'push against'.

During your adventure, I shall present to you many tools and techniques that will help you expand your perspective to where you can perceive the Systemic and Experiential Spheres. These will all work if you want them to!

The first of these is the 'Tree Plan', which is a very powerful means of defining, planning, and conducting everything from your learning experiences, to treatments, to Mastery methods, such as Essence Harvesting and course creation. The extent to which the Tree Planning system can benefit you goes way beyond the realms of Celtic Reiki and as with all Experiential dynamics is a truly integrated methodology.

To understand how a Tree Plan works, let us first examine the idea of 'shaping'; a concept that is integral to the Mountain Range of Celtic Reiki Mastery. Shapes are not only forms in the solid (spatial) world, but also in time, money, experience, etc. In fact any form of energy that is defined or parameterised in a definite way is said to be 'shaped'. One of the most effective ways to shape energy is to use an analogy, which is where you take a defined physical shape and place it in the context of the thing you want to shape. Examples of this can be found in every aspect of life, from pyramid selling, chain letters, and love triangles, to healing circles and forks in the road.

The tree has a very distinct shape that not only represents her place in the physical world (of being grounded in the Earth and reaching towards the sky, supported by the trunk), it is also symbolic of her place through time. With roots that symbolise where she has 'come from' to branches that lead to where she is heading in the future. At any given moment, the past and future are linked by the now in the form of the trunk.

We can also view the tree with the outlook of function; his roots provide water (the life-blood) and absorb, his leaves create food (nourishment) and release. The trunk transports both upwards from the ground to the air and from Grandmother Sun to Father Earth.

When we transpose the physical space of a tree into the metaphorical time and function of a tree, we create the initial concept of a Tree Plan. The purpose of the plan is to filter past and future through the filter of now (and vice versa), in addition to drawing on our abilities and knowledge to create our goals and desires (and enabling our goals and desire to hone our knowledge and abilities).

We begin our Tree Plan with the trunk. This is the point of now, the current situation, challenge, task, treatment, client, desire, etc. From this come the roots, the past, the ideas and skills we bring with us to the current circumstances, our ancestry, our foundations, the themes and life-purposes (life-blood) we want to take with us or transform in some way.

The main branches offer immediate 'paths' or directions to travel in and can also be used to represent different categories, elements, or perspectives that are decided upon now, yet lead us into the future.

The twigs and leaves are of what is to come, potential, force, energy, intangibility that is waiting to be defined, solutions, outcomes, results, and so on. You could visualise this by imagining a tree, turning it on its side and orientating the trunk, so that the roots are behind you and the branches and canopy are ahead of you.

For instance, let us say that you have a goal or desire that you wish to achieve. (This could be 'a loving relationship', 'more money', 'better health', 'inner peace', 'a new job', 'wisdom', 'happiness', etc.) Once you have decided on what it is that you would like to manifest in your life, jot this down as the 'trunk' of your Tree Plan.

The next step is to draw roots coming from the bottom of the trunk for each thought or idea you have, regarding the past or your personal history. These could be the strengths and abilities you bring to the current situation, limiting beliefs that have been instilled over the years, resources, barriers that you want to let go of, or anything that comes from the past, who you believe yourself to be, material and physical assets, or whatever you 'bring to the table'.

Once you have 'Mind Stormed' your thoughts into the roots of the tree, now create the main branches. These are based upon the context of your goal, but could contain the different aspects of your life you want to influence or contrasting elements of the goal. For example, you may decide the branches will be 'main courses of action' ('things to release', 'areas of study', 'activities to conduct', 'actions to take', and so on).

From the branches comes the canopy of twigs and leaves – these are left to your own needs, according to the individual plan, though you may choose to have twigs as 'individual actions' and the leaves as 'results', or twigs become action points and the leaves are requests for guidance and assistance, etc.

As you become conversant with the techniques and scope of the Tree Planning system, you will surely adapt the process to your own style and needs. You may, for instance, model the Fig Tree and have multiple, interweaving trunks, or the Elder, where the roots become new Tree Plans that stem from the first. The opportunities that can be derived from the method are as endless as your imagination.

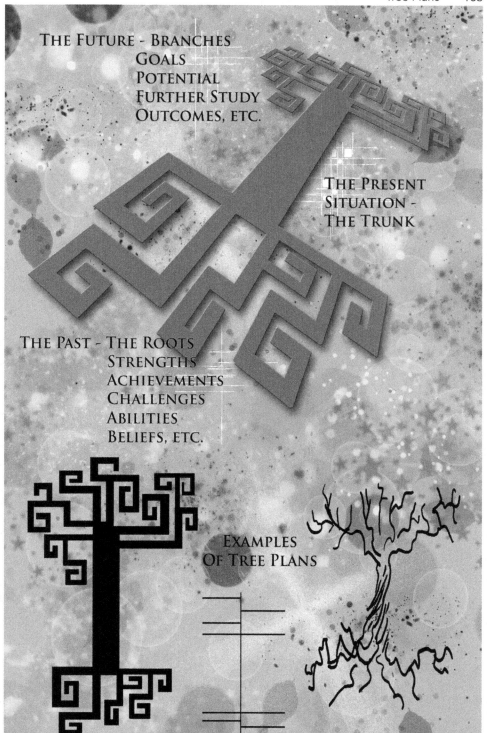

THE FUTURE - BRANCHES
GOALS
POTENTIAL
FURTHER STUDY
OUTCOMES, ETC.

THE PRESENT
SITUATION -
THE TRUNK

THE PAST - THE ROOTS
STRENGTHS
ACHIEVEMENTS
CHALLENGES
ABILITIES
BELIEFS, ETC.

EXAMPLES
OF TREE PLANS

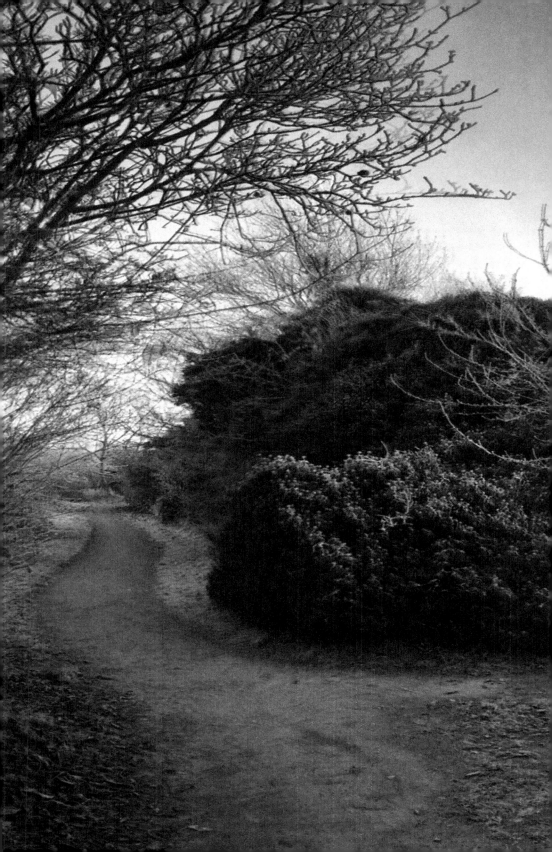

Expanding Ki & Nearth Potential

In many forms of traditional energy art or spiritual practice, the core principles revolve around some regular routine or method to increase or cultivate one's ability. The idea of Ki cultivation in Aikido or Usui Reiki and the notion of meditation are both means of increasing the connection to subtle forms of energy, and the potential of reaching higher layers of awareness.

Like any specialist, expert, or peak performer, a regular exercise or practice regime is vital to success. A marathon runner that goes for days without exercise or the opera singer that does not maintain muscle tone are not as likely to achieve their aims as those on a rigorous training plan.

The same can be said for a Celtic Reiki Master and whilst your Calibration to Celtic Reiki is a permanent feature of your awareness, it may fade without regular use and adaptation. As the needs of society and the expansion of the Universe grow, so do the requirements of your expertise.

With this in mind, I have developed a routine that you can use to enhance your abilities when working with the techniques and essences of Celtic Reiki, both from the Reiki and Nearth perspectives.

This technique can be used to create a freeform, overall enhancement of your connection, or you can choose to specialise in particular Realms, Mystics, Essences, and so on.

As a Celtic Reiki Master, the general routine will be more than adequate, however, if you want to specialise in any particular branch of Mastery (such as Realm Mastery or Mystic Expertise) then you can adapt your focus to the relevant sections of the routine.

Remember that, as with all Reiki- or energy-based arts, this is a tool that develops your grasp of core principles, as opposed to being an 'end result' in itself. In other words, this routine is a learning aid, such as water-wings or stabilisers on a bike—the main aim is to arrive at a place where you can cultivate in your own personal ways, rather than adhering to a rigid step-by-step approach. The Ki & Nearth Potential Technique:

1. Sit in a comfortable chair with your feet firmly on the floor, hands on your lap, and your spine held straight. Close your eyes and take your attention inwards.

2. State internally that you are going to "increase your Reiki/Nearth potential". (You can state either or both perspectives of energy, depending on your preference.)

3. Concentrate on your breathing for a minute or so, taking long, deep breathes. Expand your diaphragm to the sides on the in-breath and pull in your lower abdominal muscles as your exhale slowly.

4. Making your breaths longer in duration, trigger the Woodland Realm (or the realm of your choosing) and find yourself shifting into the realm perspective. You can actively Calibrate to this through your 'Core State', or simply allow it to happen naturally.

5. When in your chosen realm, you can either work with Reiki and/or Nearth in free-flow or select the essences you wish to work with. If working with essences, trigger one essence and maintain this essence for three breaths. As you inhale, trigger the essence and on the out-breath, expand the essence outwards, until it fills your perspective.

6. Once you have connected to all your chosen essences, continue to breathe, slowly, deeply and regularly. On each in-breath, imagine that you are connecting to every point of the Universe that is within your awareness and pulling the Ki/Nearth of your chosen essences from those points and into your lower abdomen. With the out-breath, imagine your lower abdomen as a ball of light that expands to every point in your awareness.

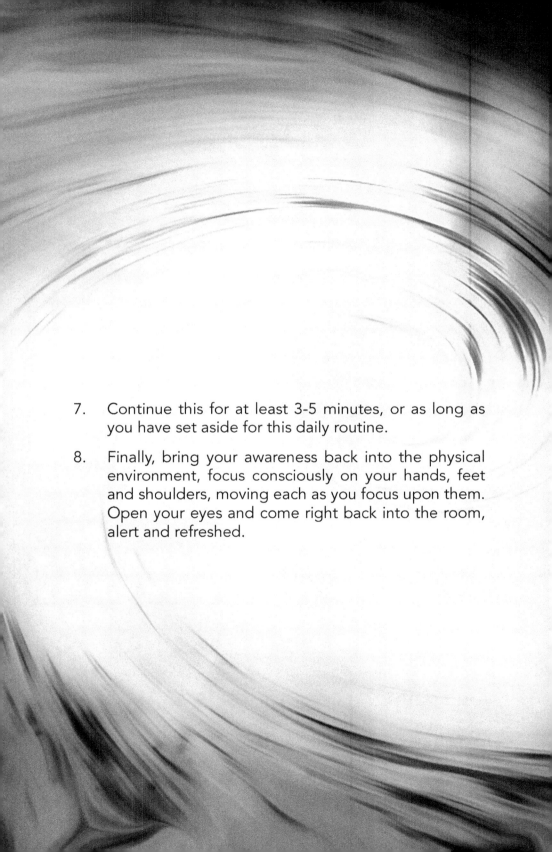

7.   Continue this for at least 3-5 minutes, or as long as you have set aside for this daily routine.

8.   Finally, bring your awareness back into the physical environment, focus consciously on your hands, feet and shoulders, moving each as you focus upon them. Open your eyes and come right back into the room, alert and refreshed.

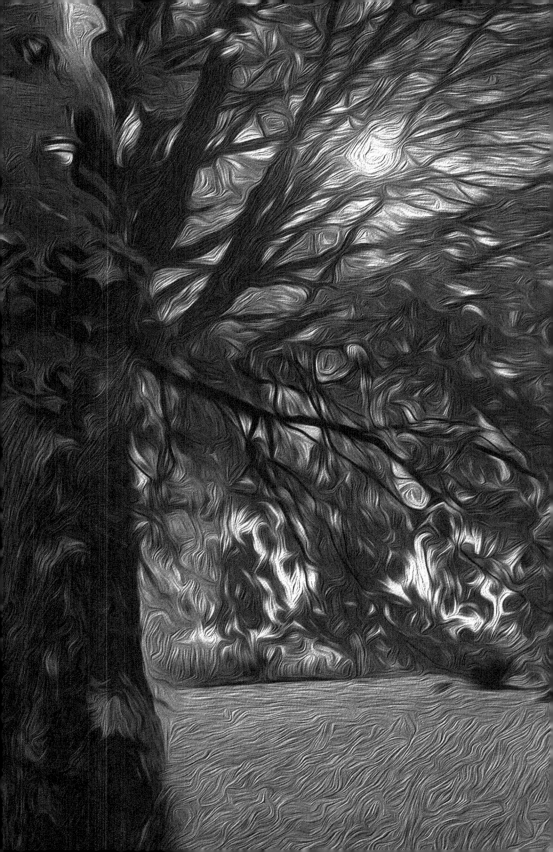

The Adventurer's Treatment Methods

In parallel to increasing your Ki/Nearth Potential, it is essential to assist the processes of Orientation and Calibration with some form of treatment. This could be as simple as initiating a self-treatment each night before you sleep, or treating yourself throughout the day at convenient times, such as whilst watching TV or even whilst doing housework!

Traditionally, a self-treatment routine consists of 'hand-positions', which are a series of positions on the body where you rest your hands to direct the flow of Reiki to that area. The Adventurer's treatment method is rather different than this, because it is more cerebral than physical. The value of hand-position-based treatments is not disputed, I feel, as the placing of hands is an excellent focus or 'statement of intent' as to where the main action of Reiki is situated (rather like pointing to direct attention).

The principle of using the mind to direct attention is beneficial, because it creates a positive habit of mental focus, as distinct from relying on physical gesture. Cerebral energy work whilst washing-up, etc. instils the ability to work from a Celtic Reiki perspective regardless of what your hands are doing and gets you into the mindset of how the physical world can be shifted by thought alone, regardless of how mundane the circumstances.

For me, this highlights the notion that joy and magic are everywhere at every moment. We often become so attached to the routine tasks or unfulfilling ways of spending time that we forget to notice the opportunities for expansion that are all around us. When you find a routine of working with Celtic Reiki, regardless of the situation, you will naturally be healthier and happier.

I do need to stress that I would not recommend using Celtic Reiki in a moving vehicle or at times when you need to be alert. This is not a question of Reiki or Nearth 'doing' anything that could be deemed dangerous – it is a simply fact that our brains need no excuse to switch off and if you're driving or operating a demolition ball at the time, it could create unwanted results!

THE ADVENTURER'S SELF-TREATMENT METHOD

1. Take several deep breaths, inhaling right into the lower abdomen and back, whilst expanding to the sides. When you exhale, keep the breath regular, continuous, and almost as if you are not breathing. This could be described as a slight muscle action and heat, without the sensation of 'breeze' or air-movement from your nose and mouth.

2. State that you are entering "Avatar State" and repeat the trigger "Adventurer", three times. If you have an internal 'image' of the Adventurer Mystic, you may wish to use this instead; whatever works best for you personally.

3. Feel an internal shifting – for me this is best described as a concertina unfolding through the centre line of my head, neck and chest. There may also be a lot of synaesthesia that you can associate with the Calibration to this Mystic. By paying attention to the synaesthetic responses, you will hone your ability to sense and 'trigger' this Mystic in the future, because these responses act as means of connecting to Mystics, realms, essences, etc.

4. Once you feel connected, focus on your lower abdomen, just below the navel and keep your attention here for 30 seconds to a minute. Then slowly, regularly, and in a controlled manner, expand your awareness down your legs, up your back, shoulders, arms, feet, and head, then beyond, out into your environment. At all times be aware of

'pulling', formication (which is a sensation like an insect crawling or spring bouncing), or resistance.

5. If you feel anything that hinders or distracts from this expansion, simply breathe into this area using an essence of your choice. To do this, trigger the essence (using the Ogham symbol and/or mantra, spoken internally, three times) and shift that point of your awareness towards the resulting perspective. For heightened effect, use your Calibration technique to match the perspective of the resistance to that of the essence. (Bring the resistance to 'Core State' and then 'travel' towards the essence, honing your 'trajectory' as you go.)

6. When the expansion happens without resistance, focus on the expansion for as long as you can. Even if you move beyond the physical walls, or boundaries of the place you are situated, maintain the expansion. Eventually your awareness will 'snap' you back into your usual conscious state. When this happens, the routine is complete.

7. At this point you can either state, internally, that "this process is complete" and continue with your day, or you can choose a new realm, essence, etc. and repeat your expansion as before.

TREATMENT OF A PAST TRAUMA

In many ways the self-treatment method will help with all forms of trauma or dis-ease, however there may be times when you want to work with some form of challenge that is connected to the past or to other people from your past. In these instances, the self-treatment method would be adequate, though for added potency use the following treatment adaptation.

1. Take a number of deep breaths, inhaling into the lower abdomen and back, whilst expanding to the sides. When you exhale, keep the breath steady, continuous, and almost as if you are not breathing,

as you did in the last treatment style. Focus your conscious attention on the past trauma or dis-ease without 'connecting' to it emotionally. If you find you are having a sudden or overwhelming emotional reaction, stop the treatment and work with the previous treatment for a while.

2.   When you have created a comfortable connection to the past situation, state that you are entering "Avatar State" and repeat the trigger "Adventurer", three times. You may want to use the internal 'image' of the Adventurer Mystic, if that suits you better.

3.   Feel the internal shifting from 'you', to 'you as the Mystic, Adventurer'. Wait a few moments for this to occur then proceed.

4.   You may be aware of the trauma 'beyond' your physical body (i.e., outside your body) or it may feel as if it is inside of you. If it is outside, expand the Adventurer out the level of the trauma, but ensure that the expansion completely encompasses you (it is in every direction and all around you, as opposed to being in a single direction). Once the Adventurer is connected to the point of focus, bring it towards you regularly and steadily, until it exists just in front of you – almost as if you could reach out and touch it with your hands. If you feel the situation internally, send the Adventurer inwards and visualise them moving the trauma to a point in front of your body.

5.   Allow the Adventurer to regard the trauma, explore it, and gain a different perspective of the situation. As this takes place, you may find that particular essences drift into your awareness or occur to you in a sudden flash of inspiration. As this happens, trigger each essence, focus on your lower abdomen, and then expand the essence from here to the point in front of you, where the trauma/situation is situated. If no essences come to mind, simply trigger three essences of your choosing or your essence of the day (as found on your online Sacred Space).

6. Continue to hold the essence at this level, though you may find that the trauma expands or contracts. If this happens, expand/contract the essence(s) to the same level. All the while gently shift the perspective of the trauma to match the perspective of the essence(s). Once there is a similarity between the issue and the essences hold this for as long as you feel necessary.

7. When ready, internally state that "this is complete" and come fully back into your usual waking awareness.

8. Use this routine regularly for each past situation, until you feel it has resolved the issue.

REALM SHIFTING

This practice will help you to move between realms with ease and speed, making the transition between different dynamics and perspectives much easier to achieve during future exercises. A Celtic Reiki Realm Master can switch instantaneously from one realm to another. The profound nature of the realms and how each realm affects you specifically, may mean that issues and dis-ease, and to a certain extent, perspective will alter how fully you grasp each realm. The more your perspective (and other factors) can transcend your personal perspective and head into Realm Mastery for each unique realm, the greater your range of abilities will expand.

The previous treatments can be completed whilst doing other activities, however, I would recommend this treatment is conducted either seated or lying down for the utmost benefit.

1. Sitting or lying down with your arms and legs uncrossed and in a comfortable position, with your back straight, take your attention to your breathing. Take several deep breaths into your lower back and abdomen, using the same style of slow, regular breath as you have done with the previous exercises.

2. With each exhalation, find yourself expanding and on every in-breath, 'fall' into yourself – not downwards, but inwards, as if flying to the centre or core of your being.

3.   Internally, say that you are entering "Avatar State" and repeat the mantra "Adventurer", three times, or use your favoured trigger method.

4.   Feel the internal shifting from 'you', to 'you as the Mystic, Adventurer'. Wait a few moments for this to occur then proceed.

5.   Choose the first realm you want to work with – such as the Standing Stones, for instance – and internally, tell the Adventurer to "shift to the (x) realm" (where (x) is the chosen realm). As you do this, be aware of any changes in perception and note any synaesthesia responses you sense. I would recommend that you use your breath to 'slow' time whilst noticing the shift. This will enable you to squeeze the maximum amount of detail from the transition into the realm and you can then use this detail to recreate an instantaneous shift later.

6.   Once you have entered the realm, use your senses to 'fine-tune' your experience of this particular realm. Does your inner vision become more colourful and sharp if you expand your awareness? If you shift your focus from left to right, do sounds become richer? How does it feel emotionally when you shape your internal position in relation to the realm? Use internal direction, position, focus, awareness, sense, etc. to monitor your synaesthesia and emotional responses and pay special attention to the experiences that seem 'better' in some way.

7.   Once you have discovered your optimum realm experience, state internally to the Adventurer Mystic that you want to go to the next realm (stating your second realm choice by name, for example, the Mountain Range).

8.   As you shift, be absolutely aware of any sensations, synaesthetic reactions and notable experiences that you can use to recreate this transition at a later date. As you practise these shifts, your unconscious mind will monitor what you are doing and remember for

future reference.

9.   Once you have completed this for all five realms, come back into your conscious awareness of your physical environment and, when you are fully awake and focused, make notes on your experiences.

ESSENCE CONNECTION FOR THE ADVENTURER

During your Celtic Reiki treatments and practices, you will soon get the 'knack' of triggering and switching between essences, simply by using the Ogham symbols and/or mantras, or by working with conscious affirmation alone. The following technique will help you to enrich the results you get from these triggers, by helping you gain a deeper insight into the effects of each essence.

1.   Before you begin, choose a handful of essences (five or thereabouts) to work with during this exercise. You may know what essences you want to work with or you can make use of the Home Experience Oracles in the realms and Sacred Space. Once you have your essences ready, sit or lie down in a comfortable position, where you will not be disturbed for the duration of the exercise.

2.   With your arms and legs uncrossed and your spine straight, align your attention with your breathing as you have done previously. Take several deep breaths into your lower back and abdomen - with each exhalation, find yourself expanding and on every in-breath, 'fall' into your core being.

3.   Internally, say that you are entering "Avatar State" and repeat the mantra "Adventurer", three times, or use your favoured trigger method.

4.   Feel the internal shifting from 'you', to 'you as the Mystic, Adventurer'. Wait a few moments for this to occur then proceed.

5.   Choose the first essence you want to work with and

internally, tell the Adventurer to "shift to the (x) realm" (where (x) is the realm associated with that essence). As you do this, be aware of any changes in perception and note any synaesthesia responses you sense.

6.   Once in the realm, trigger the essence, using the Ogham symbol, mantra, or however you prefer to shift into the essence perspectives. Feel yourself twisting, turning, moving internally, so as to orientate yourself with the perspective of the essence. Notice where or how you feel, see, hear, experience the essence and bring these sensory experiences into your entire being.

7.   When you feel completely immersed in the experience of the essence, shift the Adventurer to the realm of the next essence (if different) and trigger the next essence.

8.   Repeat steps (6) and (7) for each essence and on the final essence, return to the first once again.

9.   When you have a really good sense of the initial essence, step out of the Adventure Mystic and into your Core State. From the removed and 'inert' Core State, examine the Mystic – almost as if you are looking at yourself in a mirror – and pay detailed attention to how the Adventurer appears, sounds, seems in demeanour and body language.

10.   As you watch, the Adventurer shifts through the essences, just as you did previously, except this time, you are watching from Core State, rather than experiencing the shifts from an internal awareness. Notice how the Mystic changes with each essence and make a note of these for recording later on.

11.   Once the Adventurer Mystic has completed the cycle, step back into Avatar State and take a moment to centre yourself, before coming fully into conscious awareness and making notes.

GOAL MANIFESTATION FOR THE ADVENTURER

In the practitioner regions of the Home Experience, you will explore how to manifest goals through the three mystics and in particular the Alchemist. For the time being, though, let us investigate a routine that you can use to achieve the results and outcomes that you want for yourself. Much of the process is energetic in nature, focusing on principles, such as the Law of Attraction and positive mental attitude, however, if you work in parallel with well-defined, written goals and a proactive action plan, this will support the vibrational processes at work.

1. Write down your personal goals in a notebook or on a piece of fresh paper. For each goal, where possible, define as clearly as you can, in the present tense. So, rather than 'I want a new home', you might choose to write 'I live in a three-bedroom town-house with a corner bath and convenient access to shops and local amenities…' and so on. Clarify amounts, time scales, and as many details as you can and remember to maintain the present-tense – we often feel we have to say things as we currently perceive them to be… this is not necessary in manifestation arts.

2. Once you have your goal written down in detail (if possible 45 individual details about the goal succeeds especially well), sit in a place where you won't be disturbed and take a few moments to read over your list.

3. Then take deep breaths, close your eyes, and run through your Core State routine, as if you are Calibrating to an Orientation. Once in Core State, simply float for several minutes, breathing regularly and allowing any thoughts to glide by.

4. Using your list as a guide, pinpoint every single definition on your list, like distant stars all around you. As you internally say each defined point, see the star appear and then shift your perspective towards it. As you go to the next point, your perspective shifts again, but this time, the previous star also moves, so

that it stays in the same position.

5.   By the time you have reached the bottom of your list for the goal you are working with, all the stars that relate to the definitions you have stated should 'orbit' your Core State point in a 'fixed' position, moving in-line with your movements.

6.   The next step is to source the perspective where you have attained the goal and move towards it, treating the goal as an Orientation that you are Calibrating to.

7.   Once you are fully Calibrated, take several moments to really get a feel for how you perceive this new perspective. And only when you feel completely comfortable should you come back into the room, bringing the perspective back into consciousness with you.

8.   In the weeks to come, slip into Core State and reaffirm the manifested perspective, before bringing it back into the physical world. This can be done whilst conducting other activities which do not require focus.

THE ENCHANTED POOL

The Adventurer came to a place where the previously flat ground of the forest rippled into a crest. This small line of raised ground, sloped down into a rocky fissure; at the bottom of which was a beautiful azure pool. By the faint glimmer of light that was reflected from the rocks, the Adventurer clambered down to the pool that remained perfectly still. The night sky broke through a gap in the trees and stars were reflected from the mirror of crystal clear water.

Laying beside the pool to rest awhile, the Adventurer gazed at each star in its reflected form and wondered what the next few steps on this journey would hold. There was so much that had been learnt, not only through the words and teachings of others, but through a gradual shifting of personal perspective and the Adventurer's own expansion of wisdom. For, with everything that had been discovered, the Adventurer had realised how much more there was to discover!

It was upon thinking this very thought that a whisper voice emanated from the pool and told of what was to come... the Adventure listened, knowing that it is not the knowledge we know that creates wanting, it is what we don't know that leads us on. The more we feel we do not know, the faster we travel and the more wisdom we crave.

As the pool finished relating the many adventures to come, the Adventurer gazed upon the reflection looking back. It was no longer the Adventurer's eyes, or face, but a new visage – one of wisdom, of courage, of magic!

"Who am I?" the Mystic asked.

And an unfamiliar voice answered...

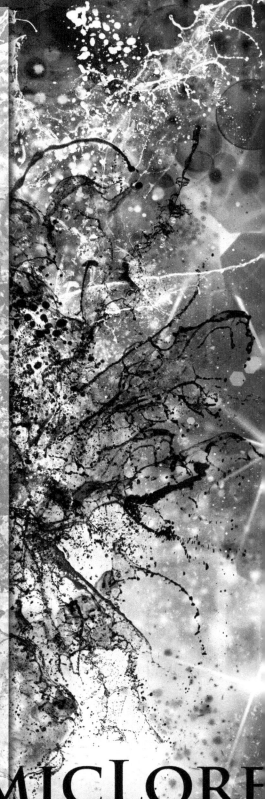

THE MORE WE KNOW, THE MORE WE REALISE THERE IS TO KNOW. AS A BALLOON FILLS WITH THE AIR OF WISDOM, NOT ONLY DOES THE PROPORTION OF AIR INCREASE ON THE INSIDE, BUT SO DOES THE AMOUNT OF AIR THAT TOUCHES THE OUTER SURFACE OF THE BALLOON. OUR REPOSITORY OF KNOWLEDGE IS THE SAME, SO IF YOU FEEL THAT YOU KNOW ALL THERE IS TO KNOW, IT IS NOT BECAUSE THERE IS NOTHING LEFT TO LEARN, IT IS BECAUSE YOU HAVE NOT STRETCHED YOUR WISDOM TO THE PLACE WHERE YOU ARE TOUCHING WHAT EXISTS BEYOND YOURSELF. TO TRULY UNDERSTAND MASTERY, ONE MUST CONSTANTLY BE SURPRISED ABOUT HOW LITTLE ONE KNOWS.

COSMICLORE

Other Celtic Reiki Books in the Home Experience:

This book is part of the Celtic Reiki Mastery Home Experience from mPowr—to enrol visit the Official Celtic Reiki Website at: www.celtic-reiki.com.

The Encyclopaedia of Celtic Reiki Essences

The Three Mystics

A Master's Companion

The Realm Master's Almanac

Realm Master: Secrets (The Sacred Wisdom of Celtic Reiki)

Discover the **Bedtime Stories of the Woodland**, now available from mPowr Publishing: the enchanting tales from the Celtic Reiki Mastery Home Experience within a single VAEO. Read the stories, hear the narration*, and interact with the characters*. Experience the wonder of the Realms anew…

*when used in conjunction with your smart phone or camera-enabled tablet device

Audio Programmes from the Author:

Synaesthesia Symphony IV: The Chorus of Creativity

Synaesthesia Symphony V:The Harmonies of Health

The PsyQ Orientation

For further information about Celtic Reiki and The Celtic Reiki Mastery Home Experience please visit:

www.celtic-reiki.com
www.mpowrpublishing.com

Lightning Source UK Ltd.
Milton Keynes UK
UKOW06f1417121117
312604UK00004B/85/P